TUBERCULOSIS
IN THE UNITED KINGDOM

A TALE OF TWO NATIONS

GW00578043

SURINDER BAKHSHI

TUBERCULOSIS IN THE UNITED KINGDOM

A TALE OF TWO NATIONS

The two nations are people born in a country with a low birth rate, such as the United Kingdom, and those born abroad in a country with a high birth rate.   Birth rate is key to the fall and rise of tuberculosis in any population.

Matador
9 De Montfort Mews
Leicester LE1 7FW, UK
Tel: (+44) 116 255 9311 / 9312
Email: books@troubador.co.uk
Web: www.troubador.co.uk/matador

ISBN 1 905237 53 7

Typeset in 11pt Stempel Garamond by Troubador Publishing Ltd, Leicester, UK
Printed by The Cromwell Press Ltd, Trowbridge, Wilts, UK

Matador is an imprint of Troubador Publishing Ltd

Lesson 7
Belief and seeing are both often wrong. We see only half the story at a time.
We see what we want to believe.
Lesson 8
Be prepared to re-examine your own reasoning
Robert S McNamara: Fog of War (Video film 2004)

I am like everyone else – I see the world in terms of what I would like to see
happen, not what actually does.
Paulo Coelho: The Alchemist

The kernel of what I want to say is that we can too easily be blinkered –
we look too easily at the obvious and then we are surprised –
Consider what do you now see?
Gerald Seymour: The Unknown Soldier

None of the ways we experience the world corresponds even remotely to the
scientific truth about it.   [Books] infiltrate and insidiously undermine the
authoritative, official version, showing it up for the sham it was.
Michael Dibdin: Medusa

Contents

Prologue

The author sought his first medical appointment, after hospital training, in a former mission hospital in Barotse province on the edges of the vast Zambezi River valley, a remote corner of Zambia on the fringes of the Kalahari Desert in South West Africa.

Barotse people live mostly in the river valley but lead a partly nomadic existence, as they have to move to firm ground when the valley becomes flooded with the overflowing river water after heavy rains every summer. The river with its thousands of tributaries provides the only means of transport. The place is best known for its centuries old, colourful ceremony of the move to land during floods, in barges, with music, dancing and feasts, described in many travel books.

A tuberculosis village was attached to the hospital. Families had to accompany patients to look after them as the hospital provided no food or other amenities such as washing soap. There were a large number of thatched huts in the hospital grounds for relatives to live in and cook for themselves and the patients. The main course of treatment was based on a cheap and readily available antibiotic. The antibiotic had to be given by injection, not suitable for treatment at home. Patients generally left the hospital as soon as they felt better, and long before the treatment was complete, which was at that time for a duration of a year. Most patients lived too far from the hospital and its satellite clinics to come for regular treatment with injections. Once discharged, usually of their own volition, patients were lost to treatment.

Equipped with a rudimentary chest X-ray machine, a microscope with common laboratory stains, and cheap and readily available anti-tuberculosis medication, the hospital would admit and treat all comers with the disease. Tuberculosis was rife. Many of the sufferers in the region had been employed as miners in South Africa. As soon as tuberculosis was diagnosed, the sick miners were sent back to their villages.

It took me years to appreciate, long after I had left the hospital and the country, that probably no one was ever cured completely with the treatment. This was just one tuberculosis treatment centre – there would be a thousand others like it all over the world. The result, over the years, was a population of partially treated people with prolonged tuberculosis infectiousness, drug resistance adding to the problem. Others have cynically pointed out that it was the cheap availability of the anti-tuberculosis antibiotic, thoughtlessly used, that did the main damage.

Poorly supervised or incomplete treatment of tuberculosis is worse than no treatment at all. When people fail to complete treatment regimens, or are given the wrong treatment, their infectiousness is prolonged rather than diminished. The bacilli in their bodies develop resistance to treatment drugs. Tuberculosis then spreads more rapidly as infected people acquire the drug-resistant strains.

Prevalence of tuberculosis was similar in developed and less developed countries before the availability of treatment 50 years ago. The change was to come later with the population explosion, wars, civil strife, famines and hunger in the less developed countries in the last quarter of the 20th century. Tuberculosis, once active at a slower pace, became uncontrolled and began to take a much heavier toll in illness and death than ever before.

Wars, famines, natural disasters and civil strife have resulted in the displacement and movement of millions of people, not only making control impossible but resulting in the rapid spread of tuberculosis as never before.

Modern drugs, however inexpensive, are of little use to countries that cannot afford them. Large areas of such countries have insufficient basic health infrastructure, where people die because of lack of not just food but also medical care.

Without treatment, people either get well naturally or die. With inadequate treatment, people with tuberculosis live longer; they eventually succumb to the disease, but in the meantime opportunity is provided for the spread of tuberculosis infection at an unprecedented rate.

Less developed countries, especially those with an increasing population, are faced with an insoluble problem. Even if drugs were available and cheap enough, health care infrastructure may be inadequate to ensure a regular supply and to monitor the disease over the lengthy period of treatment needed to achieve a cure.

Global movement of the population, mainly from less

developed countries to developed ones, brings with it an unprecedented influx of people with tuberculosis infection to countries which were on the point of being declared free of it.

It is true that the permanent solution to the problem of tuberculosis in the developed world lies in the control of the disease in the less developed one, but we must first learn to control and limit a much smaller spread in prosperous, well-resourced countries before we undertake treatment on a broader worldwide scale.

This book presents a case for the way ahead in controlling tuberculosis in one developed country, the United Kingdom.

Preface

Tuberculosis is a benign disease. Pulmonary tuberculosis, one half of all cases of the disease, is easy to diagnose, most often from the patient's history alone. Basic investigations – a skin test, chest X-ray and sputum examination – will certainly confirm the diagnosis. A three-drugs-in-one tablet regime given three times a day at home will cure the disease without fail. If detected early enough, as it must be, patients need not miss work or school. One nurse alone can manage over 50 patients at a time. There are few resource implications in managing tuberculosis in the community.

In the native-born people of the United Kingdom, 94 per cent of the population, tuberculosis has been in continuous decline for the past 200 years, at an annual rate of five per cent to start with rising to about 15 per cent at present. Transmission or spread of tuberculosis has virtually ceased. The tuberculosis we find today was acquired as an infection several decades earlier. Tuberculosis discovered now reflects a trend in infection many years old and bears no relevance to its present epidemiology. Children and adults up to the age of 50 years are epidemiologically free of the disease. Tuberculosis will self-eliminate in another 20 years or so, towards the end of the first quarter of this century.

This is the natural history of tuberculosis in the native-born population of the United Kingdom. The decline and eventual elimination is irreversible.

The natural history of tuberculosis in people born abroad in countries with high levels of tuberculosis (six per cent of the population) is different but shares one common factor. Irrespective of the country of origin, tuberculosis begins to decline as soon as people born abroad arrive in this country. The decline may be from a high level (the incidence of tuberculosis in Somalis, for example, is at least 150 times higher than in the native-born population) but it occurs in the whole United Kingdom population, regardless of place of birth. The decline is an unalterable fact, and eventual elimination in all sections of the population is inevitable.

The total number of cases may increase annually, because of increasing immigration, but the rates are always declining. No increase in rate has ever been recorded in the United Kingdom in any resident population originating from any country of the world.

All countries of the developed world share a natural history of tuberculosis similar to that of the United Kingdom. Tuberculosis will disappear in the native-born population in all these countries in 20 years or so – in some much earlier than others, but that it will do is without dispute.

This book tells you why this is so. It tells you why the United Kingdom is lagging behind the United States and what it should do to catch up. It describes the scandal of children unnecessarily developing tuberculosis and people dying from a disease easily treated.

Current means of diagnosis and treatment are adequate to ensure elimination of tuberculosis in the native-born population and if put into practice to ensure, and perhaps even hasten, its continuous decline in people born abroad in whom there is high prevalence of the disease. The problems of tuberculosis control in the United Kingdom are self-inflicted. Tuberculosis itself has long since lost the will to fight back.

Strangers at the Gate

1902: New York

The inspection process
When they landed, the immigrants had numbered tags pinned to their clothes and had to walk for about half a mile to a building where they were met by a team of doctors. The immigrants did not stop moving. Scanning the moving line for signs of illness were the US Public Health Service doctors – the most dreaded officials on Ellis Island, New York. They looked to see if anyone wheezed, coughed, shuffled, or limped. Children were asked their names to make sure they were not deaf or dumb, and those who looked over two years old were taken from their mothers' arms and made to walk. As the line moved forward, doctors had only a few seconds to examine each immigrant, checking for 60 symptoms, from anaemia to varicose veins, which might indicate a wide variety of diseases, disabilities, and physical conditions. During line inspection, those immigrants who appeared sick or suffering from a contagious disease were marked with blue chalk on their foreheads and detained for further medical examination. The sick were taken to Ellis Island Hospital for observation and treatment. Those with incurable or disabling ailments, however, were excluded and returned to their port of departure. Medical inspectors developed a letter code to indicate further examination, and roughly two out of every 10 immigrants received mystifying chalk marks. This alphabet of ailments ranged from Pg for pregnancy to K for

hernia and Ft for feet. Those suspected of having feeble minds were chalked with an X and, along with those marked for physical ailments, about nine out of every hundred immigrants were detained for mental examination and further questioning. Usually this consisted of standard intelligence tests in which immigrants were asked to solve simple arithmetic problems, count backwards from twenty, or complete a puzzle. In an attempt to deal with immigrants' cultural differences, Ellis Island's doctors developed their own tests, which allowed them to base their decision on problem solving, behaviour, attitude, and the immigrant's ability to acquire knowledge. Requiring immigrants to copy geometric shapes, for instance, was only useful for testing those who had some schooling and were used to holding a pencil. Favoured were comparisons and mimicry tests, which did not have to be explained by an interpreter, nor did an immigrant have to know how to read and write to solve them. After passing along the inspection line immigrants were waved towards the main part of the Registry Room.

At the far end of the Registry Hall, the legal inspectors stood behind tall desks; interpreters assisted them. Although the interrogation that immigrants were to face lasted only a matter of minutes, it took an average of five hours to pass through the inspection process at Ellis Island. The inspectors, wearing starched collars and heavy serge jackets, verified the 29 pieces of information already contained on the manifest sheet, firing questions at the immigrants – they asked them their age, occupation, marital status and destination in an attempt to determine their social, economic and moral fitness. Influenced by American welfare agencies that claimed to be overwhelmed by requests for aid from impoverished immigrants, the exclusion of those "liable to become a public charge" became a cornerstone of immigration policy as early as 1882. The Alien Contract Labor Law of 1885 also excluded all immigrants who took a job in exchange for passage. Together these laws presented the immigrant with the delicate task of convincing the legal inspectors that they were strong, intelligent, and resourceful enough to find work easily, without admitting that a relative had a job waiting for them. In 1917, the anti-immigration force succeeded in pressuring the government to impose a literacy test as a further means of restricting immigration. The law required all immigrants of sixteen or older to read a forty word passage in their native language. Those from Afghanistan, for instance, had to follow a series of printed commands, such as picking up a pencil and handing it to the immigration inspectors. Most immigrants, however, had to read biblical translations such as, "Your riches are corrupted, and your garments moth eaten. Your gold and silver is cankered; and the rust of them shall be a witness against you, and shall eat your flesh as it were fire" (James 5:2, 3) which was the requisite passage for Serbians. Working from 9 am to 7 pm, seven days a week, each inspector questioned 400 to 500 immigrants a day. Those who failed to prove they were "clearly and beyond a doubt entitled to land" were detained for a hearing before the Board of Special Inquiry. As immigrants did not have a legal right to enter the United States, there could be no lawyer present at this hearing, but friends and relatives could testify on an immigrant's behalf.

Unescorted women and children were detained, along with immigrants who had medical conditions and those facing a hearing from the Board, until their safety was assured through the arrival of a telegram, letter, or a prepaid ticket from a waiting relative. Furthermore, immigration officials refused to send single women into the streets alone, and would not allow them to leave with a man unrelated to them. Girls reunited with their intended husbands often married on the spot. During peak immigration years, detentions at Ellis Island ran as high as 20 per cent – thousands of immigrants a day. A detainee's stay could last days or even weeks, and accommodation was in constant shortage.

From 1900 to 1908, dormitories consisted of two long, narrow rooms, which ran on either side of the Registry Room mezzanine. Each room slept 300 people in triple-tiered bunks that could be raised, converting the rooms into daytime waiting areas. In 1906, the hiring of barges to serve as extra detention space was seriously considered. The Government allowed the construction of a new Baggage and Dormitory Building. However, this facility was not completed until 1910. In 1907 – Ellis Island's peak immigration year – 195,540 people were detained.

After inspection, immigrants descended from the Registry down the "Stairs of Separation", so called because they marked the parting of the way for many family and friends with different destinations. Immigrants were directed toward the railroad ticket office and trains, or to the island's hospital and detention rooms. Those immigrants bound for Manhattan met their relatives at the "kissing post," where many joyous and tearful reunions occurred.

The crush of immigration constantly tested the limits of

Ellis Island's facilities. Ellis Island's 125-bed hospital opened in March of 1902, and expanded in 1907 and again in 1910. Although these additions brought the hospital's capacity to 275, patients diagnosed with illnesses that warranted their detention and hospital care often numbered over 500 at a time. Many times immigrants with infectious diseases, such as measles and diphtheria, had to be cared for at city hospitals in Manhattan and Brooklyn. This prompted the United States Public Health Service to build a 450-bed contagious disease ward as well as a psychiatric ward and a morgue. "The Island is at once a maternity ward and an insane asylum," remarked one doctor. By 1911, more than 15 buildings at Ellis Island were devoted to medical care. Forty doctors, proficient in dealing with illnesses ranging from slight injuries to rare tropical diseases, staffed its hospital. During its half-century of operation over 3,500 immigrants died at Ellis Island (including 1,400 children) and more than 350 babies were born. There were also three suicides. The process of inspection and detention, and the frightening prospect of exclusion, remained overwhelming.

The immigrant screening facilities in Ellis Island were shut down in 1925.

1975: London Heathrow Airport Health Control Centre: the only port of landing with immigrant screening facilities in the world

Virginity test to prove marital status

The Immigration Officer could see that Rehana, 18, was a virgin despite her claim to have come from Pakistan to join her husband. The Officer was indeed proud of his ability to detect virgins. He ordered a medical inspector to carry out an internal examination on Rehana. Rehana was a virgin but nevertheless had been legally married, as she claimed, a few years earlier – not an uncommon practice in Pakistan.

The public conscience, which seemed to be much more sensitive than that of the government, was outraged by the revelation that some women arriving here from the Indian Subcontinent claiming to have husbands already resident in the country were being subjected to vaginal examinations at Heathrow airport to discover whether or not they were virgins, and thus whether or not their claims to the marriage state were correct.

The Department of Health saw nothing wrong with the practice, of which they were aware, but the government did prohibit further such humiliating assaults upon these women. No medical inspector has ever faced either sanction from the UK General Medical Council, the medical practice governing body, or criminal prosecution in a court of law for carrying out these acts.

1980: Dhaka, Bangladesh

Age determination by X-ray of limbs
Salim, 12, was a big boy. He looked 16. Salim's family lived in Dhaka, Bangladesh, and now wished to join his father in London. Salim, like many other children of his age in Bangladesh, had no birth certificate. The British agent in Dhaka ordered X-rays to confirm his age.

There is no "safe" dosage of any radiation, and all unnecessary exposure is illegal. Children are particularly susceptible to radiation-induced leukaemia and thyroid cancer. Bone X-rays to determine chronological age need very intensive radiation; the technique is not used in the United Kingdom. There are not even half-reliable standards to measure age available for use on immigrant children, as ethnic differences and generally poor nutrition make western measurements unreliable.

The practice was known to the Department of Health, which saw nothing wrong with it, but again, the government reluctantly ordered its discontinuance following public protest.

2005: London Heathrow airport

Inspections continue

Aisha Begum, with three young children, had travelled from her village for three nights, first on donkeys and then by bus, to reach Peshawar, Pakistan. It was to take another six days to present herself to the Health Control Unit at London Heathrow airport. There was a wait of some hours; she spoke no English and had no means of telling her anxious relatives waiting outside that she had arrived. The Health Control Unit employs no interpreters, counsellors or liaison officers. It offers no refreshments, not even feeds for babies or water to quench thirst.

Immigrant screening continues at Heathrow Airport Health Control Centre. The practice consists of chest X-rays and a physical examination less intrusive, but still harmful and no less in defiance of the United Kingdom General Medical Council rules of conduct of examination by consent, or of the Ionising Regulations relating to screening of healthy persons, setting the minimum age of 16 rather than 18 for screening with chest X-rays as defined in the Regulations.

The immigration authorities manage the Health Control Centre and allow its doctors to make some but not all decisions on its behalf. The control unit doctors inspected 150,000 immigrants in the year 2002. Arrivals subjected to further physical and psychiatric assessment numbered 1,170. Of the 700 physical examinations, 20 arrivals were sent to hospital with acute symptoms of illness, though none of them were serious enough to need urgent treatment.

A total of 57,000 chest X-rays were performed. Of these, 900 cases were referred for further investigation. Eighteen direct sputum smear positive (infectious) cases of tuberculosis were detected, a rate of 32 infectious cases per 100,000 X-rays and 12 cases of infectious tuberculosis per 100,000 inspections. One infectious case was detected every three weeks at an estimated cost of £100,000. The unit employed eight doctors, three radiology staff, 34 health control officers, and eight administrative staff. Immigration officers, security and other airport staff provided additional assistance. The Health Control Centre has asked for additional resources for its work.

Screening Tests: Predictive Values

Here I introduce concepts of sensitivity, specificity and predictive values in relation to screening tests, with brief explanations.

The sensitivity of a screening test is a measure of how good it is in identifying people who have the disease. Specificity, on the other hand, is concerned with how effective the test is at identifying people who are well.

Knowing these values, it is possible to predict how likely a test is to identify people who test positive and truly have the disease, people who test positive and do not have the disease, and those who are negative and may or may not have the disease. There is little value in a test which either identifies the disease in a majority of the people when they do not have it or significantly fails to uncover disease in those who do have it.

It is unfortunate that the two standard tests used in diagnosing tuberculosis, chest X-rays (to identify disease) and tuberculin skin tests (to identify infection) are so poor in predicting tuberculosis that the vast majority of people they identify as having the disease or the infection do not have either.

Let us take some examples.

Chest X-ray

We assume that the rate of tuberculosis in the native-born UK population is four per 100,000 population (it is less than that).

The sensitivity of chest X-ray screening in a survey published recently was 63 per cent. The number of true positives in the UK-born population is 2.52 and a false negative is 1.48. The specificity of the test in the survey was 97 per cent. The number of true negatives is 96,996.12, and the number of false positives is 2,999.18.

The positive predictive value (PPV) is the percentage of people with positive results likely to have the disease. In this example,

Number of people with positive test	= 3,002.40
Number of people likely to have disease	= 2.52
Positive predictive value	0.08 per cent

In our population of 100,000 people, 2.52 will have a true diagnosis of the disease, while 2,999.88 persons will be falsely diagnosed for it.

In the UK, new adult arrivals from countries with a prevalence of tuberculosis of 40+ per 100,000 population are screened with a chest X-ray. Let us consider an average rate of tuberculosis of 80 per 100,000 population. On the basis of the above assumptions for sensitivity and specificity, we expect that there will be 3,048 persons positive for tuberculosis; of these 2,997.6 will be false positive (50.4 true positives) for the disease.

Tuberculin skin test

Tuberculin skin test is the only method available for testing tuberculosis infection. Unfortunately, BCG vaccination also gives a positive reaction with the test. It is not possible to distinguish between the two reactions. Holland has never practised BCG vaccination. The rate of tuberculosis infection in children reflects the true rate of natural infection.

Let us accept an infection rate of 10 per 100,000 Dutch children as the norm for UK-born children. Both countries have similar rates of tuberculosis. American studies show the sensitivity of the tuberculin test in asymptomatic people to be approximately 95 per cent and specificity 99 per cent. The positive predictive value is 0.94 per cent; the number with positive tests is 1,009.40. Of these, 999.90 will be false positives and only 9.5 true positives.

The positive predictive values for the use of chest X-rays and tuberculin skin tests are too low in the UK to be of help. The use of chest X-rays in adults at ports of entry, shelters, schools, hospitals, nursing and residential homes, places of work, or in the community in general, is not valid. Outbreaks may be declared which have no basis in fact. Neither is the use of the tuberculin skin test in nurseries and schools to detect asymptomatic children with tuberculosis infection justified. Outbreaks in schools are fiction rather than reality. In a long professional life associated with communicable diseases, I never came across one tuberculosis outbreak in a school.

Introduction

The two nations in the United Kingdom, for the purposes of tuberculosis control, are people born in the United Kingdom or in another developed country and those born in a developing country. In the former, rates of tuberculosis are less than four per 100,000 population and declining fast, and in the latter from 40 to 2,000 per 100,000 population, also rapidly declining but from a much higher level. The two rates do not interact. Even within a family, a child born in the United Kingdom will carry the local rate and a brother or sister born abroad will show the higher rate.

It is important in the study of the natural history (epidemiology) of tuberculosis to understand the interactions between the tubercle bacillus and its environment (population). For a long time after the discovery of the tubercle bacillus by Koch in 1882, only two phenomena were recognised – tuberculosis as a disease, and death from it. Such events as the transmission of tubercle bacilli and the probability of acquiring infection – the most important factor in tuberculosis – were not understood.

Information on tuberculosis morbidity is voluminous and most of it is based on official records of doubtful quality. These reports do not inform us about the natural history of the disease. Events relating to acquisition of tuberculosis in native-born people (94 per cent) took place decades ago and reflect the natural history of the disease before the mid-twentieth century. Reports for people of all ages born abroad in a developing country (six per cent) reflect the natural history of that country before arrival in the United Kingdom.

The number of people becoming ill with tuberculosis who were infected abroad is increasing in parallel to the increase in the proportion of these people in this country. They, however, present a tuberculosis picture from the country of origin and not the United Kingdom where the disease eventually manifests. It is not an instance of increasing health inequality. It is not due either to ignorance of the nature and course of tuberculosis – people born in developing countries are too familiar with the disease to neglect it. Sub-optimal healthcare delivery increases morbidity and mortality from the disease. Improved training of health care workers, adherence to guidelines for treatment and use of experts experienced in managing tuberculosis will stop transmission of the disease. The speed with which diagnosis is made and the willingness to administer anti-tuberculosis antibiotics rather than adopt a "wait and see" policy determines whether or not tuberculosis will spread. Transmission is the gold standard by which to judge effectiveness of the management of tuberculosis.

The most significant, independent, risk for the spread of tuberculosis can be summarised as failure by health care workers to recognise the disease for weeks if not months and their reluctance to administer therapy to stop infection leading to disease in favour of a wait and see policy and a discriminatory approach to the management of tuberculosis.

Claims of differential responses to management on the basis

of racial or ethnic physiological variations in health and disease are overstated. Doctors ignore the dangers inherent in practising discriminatory medicine. There is no evidence that in a given environment different populations show different patterns of tuberculosis and responses to treatment.

Race, except in genetically engendered disorders, is never a good guide to disease. Tuberculosis is a disease of populations originating from areas with high rates, some of these populations are black, and some are not. Blacks of West Indian origin do not share the same propensity for tuberculosis as blacks from Africa. It is the social imagination, not the biological reality, that turns tuberculosis into a racial disease. Tuberculosis is colour-blind.

Tuberculosis once treated is cured but there is often delay lasting weeks or even months between the diagnosis of the disease and its treatment. Failure to recognise the need for early diagnosis to halt transmission is not appreciated, as is evident by the number of preventable deaths (eight per cent) in a wholly curable disease, and avoidable spread in people born in this country. Transmission of tuberculosis in this country occurs for no other reason than its mismanagement.

The blame for the failure to manage tuberculosis lies with the medical profession. Patients with symptoms of the disease are unlikely to delay seeking medical attention.

There are two reasons for this. Tuberculosis has become a Cinderella disease, important in people born abroad, but on the verge of self-elimination in the 94 per cent native-born population. Tuberculosis has become a disease on the margin, removed from the mainstream of medicine.

The second reason is the failure to understand the natural history of tuberculosis because of clouding of the issues by politicians, the media and the medical profession. How many doctors appreciate that tuberculosis is an infectious disease, wholly curable with simple medication? If we are to believe the government, media and doctors, it is a disease generated by poverty and deprivation and overwhelmingly present in asylum seekers. The truth is that asylum seekers and immigrants are as much victims of the disease as any other person born in a country where there is a high prevalence of tuberculosis. I would be surprised if even one per cent of the tuberculosis cases notified annually was reported in asylum seekers, but tuberculosis has become a political football, a proxy for the dislike of new arrivals who do not conform to the identity of the country.

London presents a special problem. Most of tuberculosis is found in the capital. It is politicised by all the main political parties – recklessly, as interference with its control may well result in an epidemic, wilfully engendered, similar to that experienced in New York a decade ago. It cost over a billion dollars to control the disease there. London may well deposit this sum as a contingency fund against the epidemic that will surely come if the nature of tuberculosis is distorted and wrong measures applied.

This book tells the modern story of tuberculosis. It is not a textbook. It is a series of interconnected topics designed to bring a fresh perspective to tuberculosis in the United Kingdom. It examines the current situation and the recent history of infection and the disease, both in this country and elsewhere, and shows the contradiction between optimum medical control and political intervention. I propose a unifying hypothesis based on the natural history of the disease and in the final part of the book set out a model for the future.

PART ONE

Pathology and Immunology

CHAPTER 1

Pathogenesis

Source

Mycobacterium tuberculosis (tubercle bacilli) is the infective agent for tuberculosis. The genus Mycobacteria also causes a variety of non-human diseases. These latter diseases, even when they occur in humans, do not spread from person to person and are not infectious. The two most common examples are *Mycobacterium bovis* (an infection caused by drinking the unpasteurised milk of an infected cow) and *Mycobacterium avis* (diseases caused by inhaling droppings of infected birds).

Exposure

Without the presence of infectious cases, no transmission will occur. Transmission (or spread) of tuberculosis requires the exposure of a person to tubercle bacilli from someone with tuberculosis. If transmission is successful, infection will take place. A source of tuberculosis in a person is required in the first place – such sources are now becoming uncommon. Even if the source is present, and exposure occurs, transmission may fail or infection not take place. In fact, the likelihood of exposure leading to infection is rare even in a favourable environment. Tuberculosis is a difficult disease to contract by chance and will not occur unless there is repeated exposure to it, in close proximity, over an extended period of time.

Exposure is not easy to define as we are all exposed to the same air space. Successful exposure will result when two or more persons are in such a confined place as to share air exchange (ventilation) within that space. The commonest source of such a space is a household unit where its occupants continuously breathe each other's air. Indeed, transmission is most successful in household contacts and is the main source of infection in tuberculosis. As a rule, exposure is confined to interaction among people of the same social group who share common amenities and interact with each other regularly. Random infection is not a feature of tuberculosis.

Factors that determine exposure are number of infectious cases, duration of their infectiousness and the number of air interactions between a case and a contact per unit of time of infectiousness. The more cases, the greater the likelihood of exposure. People who are not detected and treated promptly are infectious for a much longer time than necessary as they are discharging tubercle bacilli into the air for a prolonged period. The number of cases, duration of infectiousness and contact per unit of time cannot be quantified. Only experience with the disease is a guide to their interactive significance.

The higher the number of cases in the social group, the greater is the opportunity for exposure. The risk of exposure increases the longer the exposed person is in contact with an infectious case. One third of contacts become infected in a household where there is a sputum smear positive case. Household size is significant for transmission of tuberculosis. The average household size in the United Kingdom in the native-born population is about three. It is often much larger in households where the adults were born abroad in a country with a high prevalence of tuberculosis.

In the United Kingdom, a case of tuberculosis in a household is the main source of infection. It may be extended to the social class to which an infectious person belongs, but this is uncommon. The number of cases has an impact on transmission, as does the time for which the case remains infectious before it is diagnosed and treated. Equally, the number of close contacts per case is important, to allow the opportunity for transmission. Small households limit such an opportunity.

Patterns of social participation are a key to the exposure to tuberculosis within households. In people born in the United Kingdom, parents expose their children to a much larger extent than do their grandparents, who rarely live in the same household. The age at which people develop tuberculosis has increased and most cases of the disease now occur in the elderly. The likelihood that children will be exposed to tuberculosis has therefore much lessened, as the generation of their parents is unlikely to be infected. The disease has moved from the generation of children and their parents to grandparents.

In families originating from abroad, before social change occurs over time, children often share accommodation with their grandparents and other adult members of their extended family, such as uncles and aunts. Grandparents are actively involved in the rearing of their grandchildren. Here three generations interact closely and this social interaction results in exposure of not only children but also their parents who were born in the United Kingdom. Both inter- and intra-generations become of similar importance in contracting tuberculosis. The number of children in families who come from abroad is greater, on average, than in those born in the United Kingdom, providing a much greater opportunity for exposure to tuberculosis.

Even if the incidence of tuberculosis were the same in people born in the United Kingdom or abroad, the risk of exposure to tuberculosis would be relatively greater in the first generation immigrant children. However, such greater risk is theoretical and is not of any epidemiological significance.

Risk of disease is very high within two years of acquiring infection, decreasing over the next three years unless re-infection takes place, when the cycle repeats again. Such a risk of re-infection is low in a developed country. The risk of disease remains high in the older people born abroad, but for the younger generation, exposure is reduced by the shorter remaining life span of the older people.

Exposure does not always result in transmission, the next stage; indeed, it is much more likely that it will not take place.

Transmission

Tuberculosis is transmitted from an infectious person

suffering from pulmonary tuberculosis, producing sputum that contains tubercle bacilli. Patients who suffer from non-pulmonary (extra-pulmonary) tuberculosis cannot infect other persons, as they have no outlet for their infection. Once transmission occurs, further factors determine if infection will be successful.

Infected droplets are produced when an infectious person coughs. Only the tiniest droplets (droplet nuclei of 1 to 5 microns – less than 1/5000 of an inch) are able to float in the air currents and become airborne. A person in the vicinity, in an enclosed place, may breathe in the shared, contaminated air. Such repeated shared breathing has to be for long periods, lasting days and weeks, for transmission to be successful. The body is very efficient in destroying and dispelling inhaled contaminated air. Ten persons, on average, acquire infection from an untreated infectious person with productive cough over a year. In the United Kingdom, the time taken for infectious tuberculosis to be diagnosed and then treated is 10 to 12 weeks. During this period two to three persons become infected. In a small household, there may not be the opportunity, arithmetically, for infection to take place as only one in three persons closely exposed becomes infected over that period. The numbers are based on probability but illustrate the relative inability of the infection to spread in the average nuclear household in the United Kingdom.

In the United Kingdom, fewer than half the cases are due to pulmonary tuberculosis. Of these, only a third will have a productive cough yielding enough tubercle bacilli to be identified on direct microscopic examination. Tuberculosis is, therefore, not highly infectious. Brief exposure in casual, less intimate, occasional contact does not result in infection. Even household contacts exposed under the most favourable conditions have infection rates of less than a third.

Tuberculosis is transmitted with great difficulty, unlike other respiratory infections, and only under very restricted, favourable environmental conditions. Even when the tubercle bacilli are present in the air, they may not reach another individual, or if they do, the number breathed in may be too small to achieve transmission. Infection occurs when transmission is successful. The importance of early diagnosis is obvious. Early detection and treatment of a recently infected person will reduce disease, and therefore transmission of tuberculosis, further.

Direct sputum smear-positive patients, indicating a large volume of tubercle bacilli in the sputum, play the only significant role in the spread of infection. Patients in whom tubercle bacilli are not shown in the direct smear but are demonstrated by culture (growth in special media in the laboratory) will have much less chance of transmitting the infection to others, even to household contacts.

Infection

Infected droplet nuclei are inhaled, enter the lungs and settle in the alveoli. The sequence of events varies with a balance of struggle between the immune defences of the body and the multiplication of tubercle bacilli in the lung alveoli.

The immune system destroys the alveolar tubercle bacilli 90 to 95 per cent of the time. If multiplication proceeds, transmission is successful and infection is achieved. The infected person develops a cell-mediated hypersensitivity to tubercle bacilli four to five weeks after the primary infection. A tuberculin skin test becomes positive when this stage is reached.

Primary infection is the term used when infection occurs for the first time in a human body. The lung is the first organ involved in primary infection. Spread of tubercle bacilli occurs through the lymphatic channels draining the infection focus to the local lymph nodes. The infected site and the infected lymph nodes are together known as the primary tuberculosis focus.

In the next stage, in the majority of cases, the immune system, having failed to destroy the bacilli, is successfully able to contain but not eliminate the primary focus.

Usually no symptoms are experienced during primary infection and the person infected will not know that it has taken place. Chest X-ray will be normal and the sputum test will be negative. The only evidence of infection will be a positive tuberculin skin test.

Despite the containment of the primary focus, the immune system is not completely successful in its effort to eliminate tubercle bacilli. The bacilli are contained, but are still viable within the healed, scarred or calcified focus for the lifetime of the infected person. Reactivation may, however, take place at any time later in life.

If the immune system is not successful in containing the tubercle bacilli within the primary tuberculosis focus, the next stage is progressive primary tuberculosis.

Disease

Tuberculosis does not always follow infection. Only a small proportion of people with infection ever develop tuberculosis. Tuberculosis develops when the immune-infection equilibrium becomes unstable. We do not understand the mechanism of this disturbance.

Tuberculosis affects all organs of the body but is most likely to occur in the lungs and lymphatic tissues. Extra-pulmonary tuberculosis refers to disease in organs other than the lungs, such as the larynx, pleura, brain, kidneys, and bones and joints. Miliary tuberculosis occurs when tubercle bacilli enter the blood stream and seed most parts of the body, where they cause disease in multiple sites. The latter is a serious outcome.

It is not possible to determine whether a person will or will not develop tuberculosis. The most important risk factor is infection itself. The majority of cases that develop will do so within two years of acquiring infection. Thereafter, the risk rapidly declines and remains low but measurable for the rest of the lifetime. The latter progression of infection to disease is not important epidemiologically. The incidence of tuberculosis increases with age, which is explained both by the much greater earlier exposure and cumulative increasing prevalence of tuberculosis infection. Old age itself is not an important risk factor.

CHAPTER 2

Immunogenesis

Infected sputum droplets contain tubercle bacilli. Cough sprays these droplets into the air, which is inhaled by another person in the vicinity. The droplets containing tubercle bacilli reach the lungs and are ingested by macrophages present in the interstices of the alveoli. The presence of a foreign antigen (tubercle bacilli) triggers an immune response from the macrophages.

The defence mechanisms of the body on detecting a foreign antigen mount a counter-reaction to stop the tubercle bacilli from multiplying, and if this is successful no infection takes place.

Some of the engulfed tubercles escape destruction and begin to multiply within the macrophages. If multiplication of intracellular tubercle bacilli persists and they escape elimination from the body, a further immune response sets in to inhibit their growth. The response is a fibrous reaction around the alveolar cells harbouring the tubercle bacilli.

The tubercle bacilli remain alive but become dormant and stop multiplying within the fibrous sheath. The sheath often becomes calcified. This is the next most common outcome of the invasion of the tubercle bacilli.

The calcified focus with its inert, but live, tubercle bacilli persists for life, the infected person usually dying of some other cause. Ten per cent of the inert foci break down during the course of a lifetime, leading to reactivation of disease.

Tuberculosis infection passes through two pathological stages. In the primary, active phase (primary complex, primary tuberculosis), the infective and the immune processes attempt to establish supremacy over each other. The phase lasts about five years after which equilibrium is established and the tuberculosis infection process enters its second, dormant phase.

During the primary process, tubercle bacilli not only multiply in the lung tissues, they also often spread to local lymph nodes and even more distally to other body organs through the blood stream. In the natural course of events, primary tuberculosis is resolved by the action of the immune response, though dormant but viable bacteria persist within the healed lesions.

A much less common outcome of the primary phase is when the body fails to initiate sufficient immune response and halt multiplication. The growth of the tubercle bacilli from localised areas of the lymph nodes leads to a devastating, life-threatening spread of infection throughout the body, causing disseminated tuberculosis. This includes tuberculosis meningitis. Miliary tuberculosis results when the bacilli course through the blood to seed distant organs, the infection producing disease in all the tissues and organs of the body.

Primary tuberculosis is more common in children in less

developed countries where the intensity of tuberculosis exposes the children to infection much earlier in their life.

In developed countries, where exposure is much less common, especially in children, primary tuberculosis may develop at any age, even in the elderly if infection has never taken place earlier in life.

We do not fully understand the immunological defence mechanism, but two broad biological patterns, protective immunity and immune system-induced excessive tissue damage, are discerned which help explain the pathogenesis of tuberculosis. Whether the two patterns are the same immune process varying in degree of response or whether they are different is not certain.

A delicate balance obtains between the infection and the immune process. If the defences of the body are lowered, owing to old age and chronic ill health, or for other unknown reasons, the bacilli begin to multiply and the tissue-destroying immune pathology overcomes the protective immunity.

Once the immune-infection equilibrium (establishing a live but dormant tuberculosis focus) occurs, it is lifelong; the task of the defence forces is then a perpetual struggle to contain the infection by attempting to stop the dormant tubercle bacilli multiplying. It is successful 90 per cent of the time.

On average, 10 per cent of the dormant bacteria will reactivate during the lifetime of an infected person. The reactivation (post primary or secondary, endogenous tuberculosis) is marked by excessive adverse immune response (necrotic hypersensitivity) resulting in the destruction and liquefaction of lung tissues and erosion of the bronchial tree forming cavities in which tubercle bacilli multiply unhindered. The cavities have access to the breached bronchial tree passages and thus to the outside air. The patient becomes infectious at this stage as the liquefied lung tissues and tubercle bacilli contained in the sputum are expectorated and find an outlet to the outside air, exposing people in the vicinity to the pathogens.

The sputum brought up by a patient suffering from pulmonary tuberculosis contains a mixture of tubercle bacilli and lung tissue damaged by the immune system in its attempt to contain the infection. The immune system-mediated damage makes a patient infectious.

The immune response evolves over several years until the infection focus is stabilised. It is rudimentary in the first 12 months when infection is most likely to progress to disease. As the protective response becomes stronger, progress to disease becomes less common. After five years, the immune-infection complex reaches equilibrium and the risk of future progress to tuberculosis evens out for the rest of the lifetime. This cycle only takes place when re-infection does not occur, otherwise it too must repeat itself.

Secondary or endogenous tuberculosis, the most common form, happens when the destructive immune process is triggered in response to the reactivation of the stable infection focus. The stimulus for the reactivation is not known. Endogenous tuberculosis is never as devastating as primary progressive tuberculosis, which takes place in the complete or partial absence of a protective immune response.

In developed countries, it is the pattern for the five-year cycle to be completed, whereas it is endlessly interrupted in less developed countries when re-infection occurs repeatedly owing to the pervasive intensity of the infection, making it impossible for a stable immune-infection complex to be achieved in the secondary phase.

Tuberculosis immunity is cell mediated, differing from most other microbiological diseases such as measles, chicken pox or poliomyelitis, in which there is humoral immunity. Cellular immunity is not transferable, unlike the humoral antibodies.

While newborn babies are protected for a period after birth with transfer of humoral antibodies from their mothers, no such protection is available to babies born to mothers with tuberculosis. No age is exempt from tuberculosis.

The immune reactions are complex. The cell-mediated immune response is a double-edged sword, not only providing protective responses but also leading inappropriately to tissue-damaging immune reactions.

Tubercle bacilli do not produce toxic products – such as endotoxins or exotoxins – as do most other pathogenic bacteria. It is the defence mechanism reaction to multiplication of tubercle bacilli that leads to the injurious effects of tuberculosis. The more the cellular defence system is frustrated in halting the multiplication of tubercle bacilli, the more vigorous becomes its response with consequent damage to body tissues. It is essential to appreciate that damage to the body owing to the clinical and pathological manifestations of tuberculosis is the result of the inappropriate defence mechanism and not because of the tubercle bacteria themselves. It is a contest between the immune system and the spread and invasion of tuberculosis by multiplication of bacilli.

The pathogenesis of tuberculosis depends upon the dynamic interplay between the cell-mediated defensive immune response and the presence and multiplication of bacilli, foreign bodies in the host tissues. We have little understanding of the mechanism by which the multiplying tubercle bacilli are able to withstand the host defence mechanisms. The defence mechanism may contain the infection but it cannot eradicate the tubercle bacilli within.

The success of the immune process is indicated by the fact that 90 per cent of the infection remains dormant and the infected person dies eventually of some other cause. Immune response intervenes to limit multiplication; the host remains asymptomatic and the primary disease focus remains intact.

In a small number of infected cases, especially children, there is an uninterrupted progression from the primary infection to disease before specific immunity has had an opportunity to establish itself. There is also a marked progression to disease in four per cent of infections in the first 36 months of the primary phase, subsequently slowing down to one per cent in the following three years. Five per cent of the infections progress to disease in the first five years during the course of the primary infection.

The progression to disease then slows down considerably in the secondary phase – a further five per cent of the infection, less than 0.1 per cent annually, leads to disease in the decades following infection. It is of epidemiological importance, in view of the infection imported from abroad, that a very rapid progression to disease in the early primary period is followed by much slower progression over several decades, until old age is reached and death occurs, usually as noted from some cause other than tuberculosis.

Is there a racial and genetic difference in resistance to tuberculosis, as is often maintained in the medical literature? Are some races more prone to tuberculosis than others? Tuberculosis incidence is very high in blacks in the United States compared with all other races living in that country. Is the susceptibility to tuberculosis the result of inherent make-up or environmental factors? Or is the natural resistance the same as acquired resistance?

The consensus of scientific opinion is that there are no internal, inherent defence mechanisms that resist multiplication of tubercle bacilli. What is called natural resistance to tuberculosis is due to acquired immunity. The whole process rests on development of acquired immunity and factors that promote or retard it. Such factors are common to all races.

Hypersensitivity, re-infection and BCG vaccination

The specific immune defence response following primary infection with tubercle bacilli induces long-term protective immunity. Tissue damage is a consequence of a protective immune response. However, tissue damaging immune processes – hypersensitivity reactions – commonly recognised in well-known autoimmune and allergic conditions confer no benefit to the host. Most hypersensitive reactions are antigen-antibody reactions, but in tuberculosis cells rather than antibodies mediate hypersensitivity. Cell type hypersensitivity is slower in producing reactions than antigen-antibody reaction, hence the description, delayed type hypersensitivity.

Following infection, the body cells become sensitive to tuberculosis protein. The tuberculin skin test takes advantage of this fact. A very small dose of a purified tuberculosis protein is injected into the superficial layer of the skin. A reaction indicates previous infection. There is no correlation between a positive reaction and its size and the extent and duration of infection.

It is not yet established if the protective immune response and the tissue-damaging sensitive reactions are a manifestation of the same mechanism but differing in intensity, or are distinct phenomena. Neither do we know the correlation between immune response and tuberculin test reactions. Is the necrotic reaction the same as the hypersensitive reaction? Is hypersensitivity responsible for the body damage in primary tuberculosis and the skin reaction with tuberculin protein?

BCG vaccine works on the assumption that immune forces that prevent infection developing into disease will similarly do so in sensitivity induced by BCG vaccination. We have no scientific evidence to show that it does. The mode of action of BCG remains unknown. BCG vaccine mimics a delayed hypersensitive reaction. But is there a link between hypersensitivity and acquired immunity, or alternatively a correlation between the degree of hypersensitivity and degree of acquired resistance? It is argued that acquired immunity is a manifestation of hypersensitivity. Both coexist. Acquired immunity can remain intact after tuberculin hypersensitivity has regressed with time.

The belief persists, without evidence, that the immune system is prepared to respond positively to tuberculosis exposure in a person with primary infection rather than in someone not previously exposed. People with tuberculin sensitivity, expressed by a positive tuberculin test, are considered to have a lower chance of developing tuberculosis than those without such sensitivity, as indicated by a negative tuberculin test.

There is no evidence that pre-existing infection provides protection against re-infection, a reason for advocating BCG vaccination. Since those with pre-existing infection have escaped disease, it is argued that they have developed a better defence mechanism and are able to resist further re-infection. Recent DNA studies have shown that re-infection is as common in infected as in non-infected, healthy people depending on the intensity of infection.

Others have claimed that re-infection is necessary for

continuous sensitivity and a demonstrably positive tuberculin skin test reaction. This may be due to the fact that when primary infection does not lead to disease, the host eventually removes tubercle bacilli and the immunological memory fades over time. Again this assertion remains unproved. Deliberate reinfection through BCG vaccination would certainly put people at a disadvantage in developed countries, as natural re-infection is relatively uncommon.

There is a further problem with BCG vaccination, as we shall see in the next chapter.

CHAPTER 3

Tuberculin Skin Test

The tuberculin skin test is the only proven method for identifying infection. The tuberculin skin test reveals absence or presence of infection. Tuberculin skin test antigens are less than 100 per cent sensitive and specific for detection of infection with *M. tuberculosis*, but no better diagnostic methods have yet been devised. Interpretation of the tuberculin skin test reaction requires knowledge of the antigen used (tuberculin), the immunological basis for the reaction to this antigen, the technique of administering and reading the test, and the results of epidemiological and clinical experience with the test.

Reaction

The limitation of the test is recognised. The reaction does not distinguish between recent infection, decades old infection or an infection that is progressing to disease. The reaction due to natural infection is also indistinguishable from that due to BCG vaccination or other non-human tuberculosis antigens.

Infection is a state in which the tubercle bacilli have become established, but with no symptoms, radiological abnormalities, or tubercle bacilli recoverable on sputum culture. A tuberculin skin test becomes positive in two to 10 weeks after infection is established.

Ten per cent of infected people develop tuberculosis over a lifetime. This risk is about four per cent for the first three years after acquiring infection, one per cent in the next two years, diminishing to five per cent thereafter for the person's remaining life span.

Tuberculosis infection produces hypersensitivity to invasion of tubercle bacilli in the body. The test demonstrates the sensitisation. When tuberculin is introduced into the superficial layers of the skin of a sensitised person, an inflammatory response develops at the site, which reaches a maximum in 48 to 72 hours.

Tuberculin is prepared by producing a purified and concentrated protein fraction (purified protein derivative, PPD) from a culture of heat-treated products of growth of the *Mycobacterium bovis* organisms. Several techniques are used to introduce the tuberculin PPD into the skin. The Heaf tuberculin skin test technique was until recently the standard method used in the United Kingdom.

Techniques

1. Multiple-puncture tuberculin test (for example the Heaf tuberculin skin test) is performed by puncturing the skin of the forearm with a set of short, sharp prongs coated with tuberculin. Multiple-puncture test is easy and convenient to administer. It is no longer used in the United Kingdom.
2. In contrast to the multiple-puncture tuberculin test, the amount of antigen injected into skin is measurable

in the Mantoux test technique. It is considered a superior method for detecting tuberculosis as it provides a quantitative method of measuring infection.

The purpose of administering a tuberculin skin test is to elicit a negative or positive response in people who have been in close contact with a case of tuberculosis. Either test is suitable for this purpose.

Immunology

The reaction to injected tuberculin in the superficial layers of the skin is a delayed-type (cellular) hypersensitivity reaction, detectable two to 12 weeks after infection has been established in the body.

Knowledge of tuberculin skin test sensitivity and specificity, as well as of positive predictive values, is required to interpret skin test reactions. For persons infected with tubercle bacilli, test sensitivity approaches 100 per cent. However, false positive tuberculin tests occur in persons who have been infected with non-human mycobacterial antigens and in persons who have received BCG vaccination. These false positive reactions result in a lower specificity and a low positive predictive value in persons who have a low probability of infection. The adult native-born population has an estimated *M. tuberculosis* infection rate of less than one per cent and children born in the United Kingdom entering school have a 0.1 to 0.01 per cent prevalence of infection. Even if the test had a specificity approaching 99 per cent, testing of persons in such low-prevalence groups would result in most positive tests being false positive (due to non-human tuberculosis antigen or BCG vaccination). The specificity of the test is also dependent on the criteria used to define a "positive" test. As the interpretation is subjective, the likelihood of variability in reading a test is considerable. It would be no surprise to find disagreement between two trained people on any two-test results.

Tuberculin reactivity caused by BCG vaccination wanes with the passage of time but is boosted by the tuberculin skin test. Periodic tuberculin skin testing may prolong reactivity to tuberculin in vaccinated persons. No reliable method has been developed to distinguish tuberculin reactions caused by vaccination with BCG from those caused by tubercle bacilli.

Interpreting the test reaction and its management requires expertise and experience. The test results in themselves do not signify much. The test is widely used to predict risk of contracting tuberculosis infection in different clinical, epidemiological and pathological presentations. The esoteric science that has developed to interpret the significance of a reading is not based on fact; it is subjective and is no more precise than reading tealeaves or the palms of the hand.

For evidence-based control of tuberculosis, it is enough to know whether or not a tuberculin skin test reaction is positive when a close contact of a case of tuberculosis is tested. A positive test, despite the many reservations stated above, is accepted as positive without equivocation for the purpose of treatment. The test should not be performed if there is likely to be any doubt in its interpretation.

Despite there being a standardised technique of administration, large variations in the distribution of reaction sizes are observed. The sizes of the reactions are not always compatible with the duration of infection. They assess the individual's sensitivity to tuberculin protein; the greater the strength of the tuberculin reaction, the more likely an individual is to have the propensity for active disease, but there are considerable, unacceptable variations to this which make interpretation of reaction size unreliable.

As noted, test results can be positive when no infection has taken place and negative despite the presence of infection. The tuberculin skin test varies in the proportion of people correctly identified as infected (sensitivity), and may incorrectly identify a proportion of people who are not infected (specificity).

Further, the test results on their own cannot always be interpreted correctly. The results are interpreted in the context of another event. The same tuberculin skin test reaction can indicate a different probability of tuberculosis infection, depending on the situation. History of exposure to tuberculosis is paramount in considering the outcome of a test. The probability of a tuberculin skin test reaction being due to tuberculosis infection is greatly increased, by a factor of 10, if there is a history of recent contact with tuberculosis, as compared with no such history. When the prevalence of infection is low then its specificity is low, as is the case in the native-born population in United Kingdom. Limitations are then placed on the predictive value of a positive test result.

Tuberculin skin test reactions due to BCG vaccination

cannot be distinguished from reactions due to tuberculosis infection. BCG vaccination is the greatest bar to correct interpretation of a natural reaction and therefore to diagnostic inference. For this and many other reasons, BCG vaccination has no place in the control of tuberculosis.

Our knowledge of the significance of a given tuberculin skin test reaction is based largely on probability data derived from epidemiological surveys of patients with tuberculosis. The significance of a reaction is determined not by the size but by the clinical circumstances and the intended use of the result.

Application of the test to persons with a history of recent contact raises the expectation of the correct interpretation of a positive reaction, in comparison with persons without such a history. It becomes possible on the basis of a positive reaction to distinguish the infected from the non-infected by testing those having recent contacts.

For the purpose of interpretation of the tuberculin skin test, the population segments are divided into two broad categories, native-born and those born abroad. In the native-born population over the age of 50 years, born in the pre-treatment era, a positive tuberculin skin test is likely to be due to old infection. Such reactions are common in this group. These are not treated unless accompanying a diagnosis of tuberculosis.

On the other hand, a tuberculin skin test positive reaction is rare in native-born persons under 50 years of age, born in the post-treatment era. Discovery of positive reaction sensitivity in people under the age 50 years is promptly treated, as the infection giving rise to the reaction is likely to be of recent origin. Further, any effect due to BCG vaccination is disregarded. In people born abroad, the interpretation of the test poses great difficulty at all ages. To overcome this difficulty, treatment must always be undertaken once a decision has been made to test and a positive reaction results.

As the tuberculin test skin reaction is only relevant in the context of a host-tubercle bacilli relationship, the following American classification of tuberculosis is based on exposure history. But such a classification is subjective, not in accordance with the immunogenesis of tuberculosis. A reaction to the tuberculin skin test indicates presence of infection but does not signify disease. Disease may be present, but this cannot be interpreted from the test result. It is not the purpose of the test to extend interpretation to the quality of infection. The classification is provided as a matter of historical interest. It does not add to the understanding of the pathology of tuberculosis.

Classification of tuberculin skin test reactions

The Mantoux test uses Purified Protein Derivative tuberculin as the test material. It is the standard method of testing in the USA and Canada. It is also now adopted as the standard method in the United Kingdom.

Class 0:   No history of tuberculosis exposure.
             Any reaction to tuberculin skin test: not
             significant.

Class 1:   Tuberculosis exposure but no evidence of infection.
             Any reaction to tuberculin skin test: not significant.

Class 2:   Tuberculosis infection, no disease.
             No clinical and/or radiographic evidence of tuberculosis,
             Negative bacteriological studies,
             Any tuberculin skin test reaction: significant.

Class 3:   Current tuberculosis disease.
             Any tuberculin skin test reaction: significant

Class 4:   Old tuberculosis disease.
             History of previous tuberculosis,
             Abnormal stable radiological findings,
             Negative bacteriological findings and no clinical and/or radiological evidence of current disease,
             Any tuberculin skin test reaction: significant.

However, this classification does not add to the modern management of tuberculosis infection. The whole question of clinical management of tuberculosis is examined in Part Two.

PART TWO

Clinical Management

CHAPTER 4

Tuberculosis

Control of tuberculosis is a clinical service – treatment of an infectious disease – the success of which lies in its integration within the primary and secondary health care delivery services.

It is possible to cure all persons suffering from tuberculosis with modern anti-tuberculosis medications. Successful treatment, however, requires adequate medication, direct observation of medication if necessary and monitoring of the results of treatment.

The treatment of tuberculosis, the organisation and management of tuberculosis services, and the structure within which such services operate, is described in this chapter. Evaluation of tuberculosis control programmes and the interventions designed to bring the disease under control are also included.

To control tuberculosis, it is essential to have a clear concept of aims and priorities. The aims are to stop pain and suffering by curing the disease, and to reduce its transmission in order eliminate it. The priority in tuberculosis control is its early diagnosis and treatment.

It is worth reviewing the facts.

Pathology

Tuberculosis is an infectious disease, caused by *Mycobacterium tuberculosis* (tubercle bacilli). Tubercle bacilli enter the body by inhalation into the lungs when a person with tuberculosis coughs. Tubercle bacilli spread from their initial location in the lungs to other parts of the body through the blood stream, the lymphatic system, and the airways, or by direct extension to other organs.

Pulmonary tuberculosis is the most frequent form of the disease, occurring in over half of cases. This is the form of tuberculosis that may be infectious in about a third of cases.

Extra-pulmonary tuberculosis affects organs other than the lungs, most frequently the pleura, lymph nodes, spine, joints, genito-urinary tract, nervous system or abdomen. Tuberculosis may affect any part of the body.

Tuberculosis develops in the human body in two stages. The first stage occurs when a person who is exposed to tubercle bacilli from an infectious case becomes infected (tuberculosis infection), and the second is when the infected person develops the disease.

Infectious agents

Mycobacterium complex: The complex includes human *M. tuberculosis* (tubercle bacilli) and *M. bovis* (cattle). *M. bovis* is contracted when drinking unpasteurised milk from infected cows. It is not infectious in human beings. The term tuberculosis refers to the human type of the mycobacterial disease.

Reservoir

Humans only.

Incubation Period

The period from exposure to infection is four to 12 weeks. Infection persists throughout life unless treated. The risk of infection proceeding to disease decreases with time. It is four per cent in the first three years and then one per cent in the subsequent two years. After five years, it is less than 0.01 per cent per annum for the rest of life.

Susceptability

Tubercle bacilli are hard to aerosolise – this is necessary for them to be breathed into the lungs. The immune system is efficient in destroying most bacilli in the lungs. Even if infection does take place, not everyone develops tuberculosis. Nine out of ten people who have infection will never fall ill with the disease. Most infection lies in a dormant state in the body throughout life. We do not understand who will develop disease because as yet we do not understand the state of dormancy.

It is estimated that each untreated infectious person infects about 10 people in a year and of these 10, one infected person will develop disease.

No age is exempt from tuberculosis. The risk of infection is related to the degree, frequency and intensity of exposure. It is not related to genetic or other host circumstances, or environmental factors. The first 12 months of infection are the most hazardous with two to three per cent resulting in disease. Reactivation of infection accounts for the disease in adults in the native-born segment of the population.

Infectiousness

Infectiousness is present as long as tubercle bacilli are present in the sputum. Treatment rapidly reduces the tubercle bacilli load and their presence in the sputum within a few days. Risk of transmission, even to close contacts, is reduced to a minimum. Tuberculosis ranks low among infectious diseases in infectiousness per unit of time of exposure, and provided diagnosis of infectious cases is promptly made, the chance of even a close household contact becoming infected is less than 10 per cent in four weeks. The average delay in diagnosis is two to three months, which will result, on average, in one to two new cases of infection for each index case. If the rate of tuberculosis is four per 100,000 native-born population, the rate of infection will be five to 10 per 100,000 (0.02 to 0.04 per cent) native population.

Transmission

Persons with infectious tuberculosis in whom the tubercle

bacilli are so numerous as to be seen on direct microscopic examination of sputum specimens (smear positive cases) are the most infectious. Those in whom tubercle bacilli cannot be seen directly under the microscope (smear negative cases) are very much less infectious and the severity of their disease is less than that of the smear positive cases. Extra-pulmonary cases are not infectious.

The infectious person expels tubercle bacilli into the air in minute droplets when coughing, laughing or sneezing. The droplet nuclei carrying the tubercle bacilli remain suspended in the air for a few hours. A person who shares an enclosed space may inhale these droplet nuclei. If the tubercle bacilli establish themselves in the lungs and begin to multiply, infection has occurred.

Exposure to the tubercle bacilli and infection is greatest among people in close and prolonged contact with an infectious case, such as those living in the same household. The chance of becoming infected from a limited and occasional contact with tuberculosis, in schools or place of work, is rare.

Progress of infection

Among people who do become infected, 90 per cent will never become ill with tuberculosis. The tubercle bacilli remain dormant within the body and their presence is indicated only by a positive reaction to a tuberculin skin test. Infected persons who do subsequently develop disease are most likely to do so in the period immediately following infection, but the risk, though small, continues throughout the remainder of their lives.

Diagnosis

Symptoms
The symptoms of pulmonary tuberculosis are persistent cough with sputum production, shortness of breath and chest pain. Symptoms common to all forms of tuberculosis are loss of appetite and weight, feeling of illness (malaise) and tiredness (fatigue), night sweats and fever.

A person presenting with these symptoms who is in contact with a person with tuberculosis is most likely to be suffering from tuberculosis.

Symptoms of extra-pulmonary tuberculosis depend on the organ involved. Chest pain from pleurisy, the presence of enlarged lymph nodes, and angular deformity of the spine are the most frequent signs of extra-pulmonary tuberculosis.

Tuberculosis is most frequently found among persons who present themselves to a doctor with symptoms suggesting tuberculosis and are living in the same household as a person with tuberculosis. In addition, an abnormality on a chest radiograph that has the appearance of tuberculosis may lead to the initial presumptive diagnosis of tuberculosis.

Tuberculosis will be detected most efficiently where doctors are alert to the symptoms suggestive of the disease.

Bacteriology

Every person suspected of harbouring tuberculosis must have an examination of sputum to determine whether or not they have infectious tuberculosis. The examination consists of microscopic examination of a specimen of sputum stained by the Ziehl-Neelsen method (smear microscopy). If tubercle bacilli are detected, the person is said to have sputum smear positive (infectious) tuberculosis.

Whenever tuberculosis is suspected, three consecutive daily specimens are collected for examination by microscopy. It is found that of those persons who are positive, approximately 80 per cent are demonstrated on the first examination, 15 per cent on the second, and five per cent on the third.

Radiology

Diagnosis by means of radiographic examination in persons suspected of tuberculosis is not always reliable. Abnormalities identified on a chest radiograph may be due to tuberculosis or to other conditions. There is a specific appearance for tuberculosis on the radiograph. Chest radiographs are generally more helpful in those persons who are not sputum smear positive but are considered to be suffering from tuberculosis.

Tuberculin skin test

A tuberculin skin test is performed to help in the diagnosis of tuberculosis infection. The interpretation of a test result is often difficult, as a positive test may be caused by factors other than by tuberculosis and a negative test does not always rule it out.

Diagnosis in children

Diagnosis of tuberculosis in children is difficult. In the majority of cases, childhood tuberculosis is a mild disease that heals of its own accord, even without treatment. The exceptions are disseminated tuberculosis and tuberculosis meningitis, rare forms of serious tuberculosis in children. Children with tuberculosis infection are always treated to prevent the disease and the subsequent development of tuberculosis from reactivation of their past infection in later life. Only a very small proportion of children have smear positive (infectious) tuberculosis. In determining a diagnosis in children, note is made of

- history of contact with a case of infectious tuberculosis in the same household
- and/or abnormal chest radiograph showing unilateral lymphadenopathy
- and/or shadows in the lung field indicating infiltration
- and/or positive tuberculin skin test.

Any child under five years of age in contact with a smear positive case and with signs or symptoms suggesting tuberculosis must be treated for the disease. Those without signs or symptoms of disease but a history of family contact are given preventive chemotherapy. There is no place for a wait and see policy in suspected children.

Treatment

If the diagnosis of tuberculosis is made at an early stage of the disease, it is possible to cure all cases and prevent spread. Chemotherapy is the most efficient means of preventing the spread of tubercle bacilli. The requirements for chemotherapy are a combination of anti-tuberculosis medications to prevent the development of resistance, prescribed in the correct dosage, and taken regularly for a fixed period, to prevent relapse of the disease after completion of treatment.

Treatment is commenced as soon as a clinical diagnosis is made. No delay should occur while waiting for laboratory or other results. The clinical suspicion of tuberculosis should dictate action. Treatment can always be stopped if the diagnosis proves incorrect, but delay can result in the progress and spread of the disease.

Treatment of tuberculosis starts with an intensive medication phase. An initial course consists of a combination of medications effective in eliminating tubercle bacilli and in minimising the influence of tubercle bacilli that are resistant to medications. The intensive phase is given for a minimum period of two months. The intensive phase is the most important part of the chemotherapy. The patients are free of the tubercle bacilli at the end of this period.

The second phase is the continuation phase. This does not require as many medications but does require a sufficient duration to ensure success. This is usually four months. The total duration of medication is six months. The patient is permanently cured at the end of this phase. Relapse is unlikely.

It is vital that the person takes the total quantity of medication prescribed. To ensure that this occurs, frequent and careful supervision is essential. It may be occasionally necessary for a health care worker to observe that the person swallows every dose of the combination of medications given. This will require the person to be present for direct administration on an agreed basis for the period during which therapy is given.

Otherwise medication is usually given in monthly supplies for daily self-administered intake at home. This limits the duration of time required to attend the health service for treatment, freeing the person to return to normal daily activities after the initial intensive phase. When the person has completed the prescribed duration of treatment, the medications are stopped.

There are an agreed number of medications currently available for the treatment of tuberculosis. The most important are isoniazid, rifampicin, pyrazinamide, ethambutol, and thioacetazone. The medications are available in combined preparations, so that it is only necessary to take one tablet of combined treatment at a time. The medications, by universal agreement, should be available to the patient only through tuberculosis programmes. There is international agreement on the recommended dosage of each anti-tuberculosis medication, which is calculated per kilogram body weight of an individual.

Infectiousness following treatment

Treatment is effective in rapidly diminishing the infectiousness of a person with tubercle bacilli. This is because the medications reduce the number of tubercle bacilli in the sputum, and the person's cough subsides, resulting in fewer tubercle bacilli expelled into the air. In most settings, no special precautions for preventing the spread of infection need be taken once the person is on treatment. The best prevention is to ensure that the medication is being taken regularly. The quality of the care given to persons and the thoroughness with which treatment regimens are followed are important determinants of success. Poor treatment increases the number of infectious cases in a community.

Drug resistance

Resistance to medications is a problem. Populations of tubercle bacilli always contain some mutants naturally resistant to medications – the resistant bacilli are always selected when less than adequate medication is used. This occurs because only the tubercle bacilli susceptible to the medication are killed, leaving the resistant ones to multiply. When the tubercle bacilli in a person are resistant to all but one of the medications given, the treatment has the same result as when a single medication is given alone. There are two important types of resistance to medications in tuberculosis.

Acquired or secondary resistance is due to incorrect treatment; for instance, treatment with a single medication in persons with tuberculosis (monotherapy), or administration of medications to a person harbouring tuberculosis tubercle bacilli resistant to all but one of the medications given.

Primary resistance occurs when a person develops

tuberculosis after being infected by another person who has resistant tubercle bacilli. Tubercle bacilli with resistance to the two most important medications, isoniazid and rifampicin, at least, are termed "multi-drug-resistant". Primary resistance is rare and is usually imported from abroad.

Treatment of infection (preventive therapy)

Those who live in the same household (contacts) with a person who is sputum smear positive are exposed and have a very high risk of developing tuberculosis infection. A child in the household who is under five years of age and who has symptoms that suggest tuberculosis is treated even when the diagnosis is in doubt. All other children under five years of age, whether infection has been established or not, are given preventive chemotherapy. Previous vaccination is disregarded.

Preventive therapy is the treatment for those infected with tubercle bacilli (tuberculosis infection) who do not have the disease (tuberculosis). The infection is identified with a tuberculin skin test. The risk of developing tuberculosis in those who are tuberculin skin test positive is low unless the infection was acquired recently. Preventive therapy in such persons prevents the development of tuberculosis.

The anti-tuberculosis drug isoniazid is used for preventive treatment for a period of six months. The most important group needing preventive therapy comprises children under the age of five years who are living in the same household as a newly discovered tuberculosis sufferer. The chance that such children have been infected is high, as is the chance of the development of tuberculosis following infection.

Follow-up

Because tuberculosis treatment is prolonged, great care is taken to ensure that the treatment is taken as prescribed by all persons needing it.

Cooperation with treatment

Successful treatment requires that the patient understands what is happening. When a person understands the nature of the disease and its treatment, he or she is more likely to follow the procedure required to achieve cure. The relationship developed between the person and the caregiver is key to achieving success in treatment. It needs investment of time and energy.

Monitoring progress during treatment

Bacteriological follow-up examinations in smear positive persons are the most important means of assessing progress. After two months of intensive phase treatment, the sputum in these persons must be examined. Those found to have no tuberculosis tubercle bacilli are allowed to start the continuation phase. The microscopic examination is repeated at five months. If the result is negative, treatment is continued for one final month. If tubercle bacilli are identified, treatment failure is recognised and a re-treatment regimen commenced.

The total duration of treatment is always six months for daily regimen or 12 months for intermittent treatment. Persons who occasionally miss treatment should have the time missed added to the duration originally planned.

Organisation of delivery of tuberculosis services based on recommendations by the World Health Organisation

Because tuberculosis prevention is dependent on good quality medical care, the organisation through which this care is given is an important factor in achieving success.

The responsibility for activities is organised in the form of a local Tuberculosis Control Unit based in district general hospitals. It coordinates with the local primary care, microbiological and radiological services. It has on average a minimum of 150 patients on its register at any one time.

The local units are linked to a National Tuberculosis Unit. The National Unit is responsible for all tuberculosis activities in the country. The National Tuberculosis Unit plans, implements, monitors and evaluates the national tuberculosis programme. Training of health care workers is an important responsibility.

To achieve their aims, local services must be integrated within the general health services to make certain, firstly, that all new cases arising from transmission of infection or already infected are identified promptly and cured, and secondly, all contacts who have become infected, or are at risk of infection, especially children, are identified and treated.

The programme must be adapted to the local needs taking note of the characteristics of the population and the availability and accessibility of health facilities. It must provide for the diagnosis and follow-up of tuberculosis based on sputum smear microscopy, chest radiology, and treatment – monitoring through proper recording and reporting of activities. In order to maintain a good quality of service, a system of training and supervision must be in place to support the tuberculosis control programme.

Laboratory service

A well-functioning laboratory is the first requirement for successful management of tuberculosis. In principle, the microscopy centre should be located at the same site as the treatment centre, for if the diagnosis is not made reliably and quickly and if follow-up of treatment is not trustworthy, all other activities will be affected. The aims of the laboratory service with respect to tuberculosis are confirmation of diagnosis, monitoring of treatment of infectious cases, and surveillance of the tuberculosis situation in the population.

Quality assurance of all laboratory investigations is essential if the tests are to be meaningful and useful in the care of the person. Because sputum smear microscopy is so important, quality assurance is an indispensable component of any tuberculosis programme. A regular system of quality assurance must be part of the supervision process, and re-training of technicians who perform their duties in a deficient manner must be undertaken.

Monitoring of care

The adequate care of cases requires that records be kept on each person, with periodic reporting of the case findings and results of treatment. This is essential to ensure that the person is correctly treated. In addition, the information that is routinely collected and reviewed allows problems that may arise with the management of the patients and the system to be identified. The documents used to record and report the care of the persons must be simple, clear and kept to the necessary standard that is required for adequate care.

If someone is designated a tuberculosis case, a personal identity card is completed and kept by that person. At the same time, a tuberculosis treatment card is made and is kept at the health service where the person receives treatment. The information from this card is entered into the tuberculosis register within the unit where the person's care is managed.

Reporting of the case findings and the results of treatment permits the tuberculosis activities to be evaluated and allows early identification of problems in the health services. The reports are used primarily for planning future activities and are recorded in a Tuberculosis Register within a period agreed upon. They also provide information concerning the number of new cases of tuberculosis classified by age, category, and sex. At the time the report on the case is completed, a report on the results of treatment is also prepared.

Evaluation

Evaluation of tuberculosis requires scrutiny both of the tuberculosis situation and of the control measures (interventions) applied. Evaluation of the control measures is accomplished through the reports on case findings and on treatment.

Targets for control measures are established at local levels. A comparison of the results achieved with the targets that have been set forms the basis of evaluation of the control measures applied.

The most important evaluation is the regular review of the results of treatment. The proportion of all cases that have defaulted from treatment reflects the organisation of the services. The only way to achieve acceptable results (the ultimate target of the treatment programme) is by reducing the number of persons who default. This indicates whether people find the service accessible and appropriate. This is the most important target. Another outcome to monitor over the course of time is the proportion of cases that are smear positive at five months or more after starting treatment (treatment failure) – this is an indication of the efficacy of the regimen utilised and indirectly suggests the level of resistance to medication.

The regular review of reports allows treatment activities to be evaluated. Progress in approaching the targets can be determined by comparing various geographical regions of a country to identify problem areas. Trends in the results of treatment (both positive and negative) can be defined in a single location, indicating the quality of care in that location.

Evaluation of a tuberculosis programme (epidemiological surveillance) is important to enable planning and budgeting and to adjust the programme in relation to the challenges identified. Several epidemiological indices have been utilised for measuring the extent of the tuberculosis problem in a given population.

The rate of reported smear positive cases is used when reporting of smear positive pulmonary tuberculosis cases is complete. The completeness of notification is dependent upon the coverage of the diagnostic service (sputum smear microscopy), its reliability, and upon the efficiency of the reporting system. This is the most practical means of surveillance and its accuracy and completeness should have high priority among surveillance activities. Prevalence of smear positive pulmonary tuberculosis records shows the number of infectious cases in a community at a given point in time.

Conclusion

Tuberculosis can be controlled. The reason why this is possible is that the source of the infection is almost exclusively a person who is ill with the disease and who is easily identified. The rate of spread of infection is reduced if the infectious cases are identified and treated. The transmission of tubercle bacilli is relatively inefficient, so that any reduction in the number of sources of infection and the period of time each is infectious will improve the epidemiological picture. The tools required to carry out the tasks (sputum smear microscopy, basic radiology, and chemotherapy) exist and can be applied efficiently.

Poor treatment of tuberculosis spreads infection to uninfected persons and increases the number of sources of infection. It keeps alive a person who is not cured and who would otherwise have died, thus spreading the disease.

Poor treatment has another, very serious, consequence. Persons who are treated for tuberculosis but fail to be cured are at a high risk of developing resistant tuberculosis and transmitting it to others.

Finally tuberculosis is controlled successfully only in the context of a dedicated local tuberculosis programme. Such a programme must operate within the routine health services. The United States has shown that when the recommended programme is put into practice tuberculosis control is rapidly achieved, and this is discussed more fully in Chapter 10. First, though, I would like to look in more detail at other aspects including, in the next chapter, the particular case of children and tuberculosis.

CHAPTER 5
Tuberculosis in Children

Children in the United Kingdom are normally infection free. Infection indicates recent contact with a case of tuberculosis. Tuberculosis in children is evidence of inadequate or no treatment. The occurrence of tuberculosis in children provides important information about the spread of the disease. When a child has tuberculosis, we learn that it was transmitted recently, that the person who transmitted the infection to the child is most probably still infectious, and that other adults and children in the family have also been exposed to the disease.

Children born abroad may bring infection into the country with them. It is not possible to know if the infection was acquired recently or whether it had been present for some time. Such infection, if detected, is promptly treated regardless of its antecedents or of a previous BCG vaccination. Treatment of infection is the cornerstone of tuberculosis control. Children develop tuberculosis rapidly after infection. Children are more prone to developing life-threatening forms of tuberculosis than adults. Tuberculosis causes death from meningitis and disseminated disease in children. Death from the disease in children indicates failed tuberculosis control.

Tuberculosis in children is linked to a case in an adult in the family. Each case of tuberculosis in a child is a failure of management as it is so easily prevented. It is a measure of recent transmission of the disease, because those children who develop tuberculosis tend to do so rapidly, usually within weeks after initial infection has occurred. As a result, the rate of the disease in children is an indicator of the current rate of transmission within the population. An increase in tuberculosis in children is a harbinger of its future resurgence in adults. Tuberculosis in children is a measurement of future infection in adults who by re-activation develop it from infection acquired during childhood. Treatment of childhood infection would prevent adult cases in the future.

Absence of tuberculosis in children indicates failure of transmission. This in turn indicates good control of tuberculosis in the population. Failure of tuberculosis in children is a better index of control of tuberculosis than its incidence. In immigrants, however, infection may have been acquired in the country of origin. Most of the tuberculosis in children found in the United Kingdom is in those born abroad. Disease from infection acquired abroad is inevitable and cannot be prevented. Prevention of its further transmission, however, is an objective of a control programme.

Diagnosis of tuberculosis in children is difficult. Children do not produce sputum for examination. A history of contact with a person with tuberculosis, with or without the triad of an abnormal chest X-ray, physical signs, and a positive tuberculin skin test, can be enough for the diagnosis to be made in children. History of contact may alone provide a diagnostic clue to tuberculosis. It is most often the only clue.

Treatment of adults only will have a minimal impact on tuberculosis in children, as the latter may already be infected. Even small increases in cases found and their treatment will have an influence and cause an eventual decline in the severity and amount of childhood tuberculosis. Treatment of children with tuberculosis exposure and infection will prevent disease.

Children who are exposed to tuberculosis in the family should always receive treatment, even if there is subsequent evidence of failure to establish infection. The treatment of exposed children should be standard practice in developed countries and the failure to treat children at this stage inevitably leads to cases of preventable tuberculosis in the future. The tuberculin skin reaction may not become positive for as long as three months. However, the incubation period of disease, particularly life-threatening forms, may be less than three months so that disease occurs before the tuberculin skin test becomes positive. Exposed children are placed on medication until a repeat tuberculin skin test three months later can prove that the child is not infected – the medication can then safely be discontinued. The rate of infection in exposed children is high. Since children who develop tuberculosis tend to do so rapidly, the recently infected children are most likely to develop tuberculosis disease within a short time.

Children with symptoms who are family contacts of tuberculosis sufferers are treated for the disease. The rationale for treating symptomatic children is simple. Because anti-tuberculosis medication is well tolerated by children, the risk of adverse reactions is low, so the risk benefit ratio favours treatment. If the child is infected, treatment will prevent development of disease. If the child is not infected, there is little harm as the medication is safe. If the child has early symptomatic disease, the disease will be cured.

Children, ideally, receive medication under direct observation therapy (DOT). DOT is not simply the provision of medication, it is a package of services designed to support the patient and the family during treatment. Making sure that the other children in the family do not develop tuberculosis is a fundamental part of this support and an essential element of the DOT programme.

Childhood tuberculosis will be missed if attention is not paid to families that have recognised adult cases. There is also the danger of misdiagnosis as the clinical and physical findings of children with tuberculosis are rarely specific. The most powerful piece of information pointing to the diagnosis of tuberculosis remains recent exposure to a case of tuberculosis in an adult. Without contact investigation, children with tuberculosis infection are diagnosed much later, after they have become symptomatic. This leads to much higher rates of morbidity and mortality than if steps to diagnose and treat tuberculosis are taken in time.

There are only two ways that a child acquires tuberculosis infection: within a family in this country, or in another country in which the child was born. It is not possible to tell if a child born in another country acquired the infection in the resident country or abroad. This may be of epidemiological significance, but it is not important when considering treatment. If a child is a close contact of a case of tuberculosis, the child must be treated. A family-centred service will find and treat all recently exposed and infected children so that their disease is prevented or treated early. The DOT is used to prevent serious outcome of the disease and eliminate a future reservoir of tuberculosis infection. Tuberculosis in children should be treated only by doctors with experience of treating such an illness, because of the highly subjective nature of the diagnosis of the disease.

CHAPTER 6

WHO Policy of DOT: A Strategy Doomed to Failure

As we have seen, control of tuberculosis depends on its treatment. Treatment cures tuberculosis. Failure of tuberculosis programmes to reduce its incidence in less developed countries led to a review of World Health Organisation (WHO) policy on control of tuberculosis in 1994.

The revised policy emphasised improvement of tuberculosis cure rates of individual patients rather than the number of people treated for tuberculosis. Effective individual treatment was the key, to be achieved by direct observation of patients taking their treatment. Principles of integrated care were formulated, but the essential underlying factor was that the treatment must be offered under direct supervision, hence the name of the programme, DOT (direct observed therapy).

The WHO has mobilised resources in less developed countries to control tuberculosis under its DOT strategy. It now claims that this system has revolutionised treatment of tuberculosis in less developed countries and actively promotes the policy worldwide. No alternative programme is offered.

The presumption was that it was the inability to follow

treatment which resulted in the failure to cure tuberculosis. Patients could not be trusted to take three tablets a day on their own. It was to drive the point home that the policy directed patients to take their medication under direct supervision of a health care worker. Readers will understand the enormity of this step if they consider a scenario where every patient in the United Kingdom suffering from a chronic illness – diabetes, heart disease, hypertension and rheumatoid arthritis are examples – received medication under supervision.

Readers who have read this book so far will no longer be surprised to learn about the lengthening series of man-made obstacles making an eminently treatable disease untreatable. The DOT strategy is one of them. Unfortunately, more examples are to follow.

The availability of anti-tuberculosis medication has not proved a boon in less developed countries. They are unable to treat the disease because of lack of an organisation to deliver the service, inadequate control and cost of drugs. Very often patients stop taking treatment as soon as they feel better. The symptoms tend to subside just a few weeks after starting treatment, even though the disease is still active in the body. Anti-tuberculosis medications are widely available without restrictions in the market in less developed countries. Most often, however, patients can only afford partial treatment if they have to pay for the drugs, as is often the case.

The result is that within a decade of the availability of anti-tuberculosis antibiotics, poor treatment resulted in prolongation of infectiousness in partially treated people and drug resistance owing to the improper use of medications, without a cure being achieved, as would be the case with every treated patient in a developed country.

About this time, New York, USA, suffered the largest epidemic of tuberculosis in the modern world in people who had no access to medical care. The United States found itself in a position where it was now prepared to control the disease, but had no organisation to do so. It decided to follow the patients and treat them on the spot wherever they could be found. It helped to bring tuberculosis under control at a huge cost, but was not an example of good delivery of a health service because other health needs remained untouched. It cost over a billion dollars to bring the epidemic to a halt, a sum exceeding the health budgets of most poor countries in Africa.

The United States then made virtue of the necessity to go to the patient to treat tuberculosis as the gold standard for control. It suggested that the outbreak was not the result of lack of treatment but was because the ill people were not taking their medication. As an example of blaming the victim, it could not be bettered.

The WHO found great consolation in this policy. It was not really to be blamed for failure of tuberculosis control in less developed countries. Its new strategy was based on the fact that tuberculosis control failure in less developed countries was due to the failure to accept treatment, hence the emphasis on overcoming that problem in the title of its programme. The WHO asks donors of aid to tuberculosis programmes to insist on the DOT strategy being adopted so as to be eligible for help. It regards direct observation treatment as the biggest health breakthrough in the control of tuberculosis. While there have been major modifications to the WHO programme launched in 1995 direct observation remains the core to the current WHO strategy. The energy which goes into insisting that direct observation is essential and non-negotiable has its opportunity costs and drawbacks when other alternative strategies are not considered.

There is no argument that resources, medication, political support and active management of programmes help improve control of tuberculosis. But the WHO is not concerned whether less developed countries are able to implement the policy on a national level. I know of no example of a developed country that has either adopted this approach or could even afford to do so. This includes the United States. As long as those who receive treatment are cured, the WHO is satisfied and will support local programmes irrespective of whether there is a viable national DOT programme to control tuberculosis in the rest of their country. DOT takes health care workers away from other essential tasks such as control of malaria or HIV/AIDS. The onus is on governments to provide resources and organisational requirements for the range of support measures necessary for patients with tuberculosis to be able to adhere to treatment under observation. It is not surprising that DOT programmes, though much talked about, have still to influence global tuberculosis a decade after their introduction. There is more tuberculosis in the world now than there was when the DOT strategy was launched.

DOT programmes are often of such poor quality that

patients prefer to remain without treatment. Ironically, direct observation reduces adherence as it places an immense economic and social burden on patients who have to abandon families and employment in order to go to a specified clinic to take medicine under supervision.

By far the worst outcome of DOT is the unwarranted assumption that patients cannot be trusted to take their medicine without observation. If the purpose of DOT is to promote adherence to treatment, then lack of trust in patients is not going to achieve success in the long term. Well-conducted programmes promote adherence. This is indeed the experience in developed countries. Direct observed therapy may be necessary in a small proportion of patients, especially children, who find it difficult to follow the treatment regime for a prolonged period, but it certainly is not the method to be adopted to treat all patients. Even the United States, which vigorously promotes DOT for less developed countries, does not follow its own advice because most people with tuberculosis are compliant with treatment – DOT programmes would be too expensive even for the richest country in the world to be able to afford them.

It is not surprising that independent studies show no advantage of direct observation over self-treatment at home in relation to cure. The less developed countries are saddled with an expensive and impracticable plan. Many countries prefer to finance their own programmes rather than to rely on donors who insist on DOT. More importantly, adoption of a DOT programme affects care of patients with other illnesses – such as malaria – which are in just as much, if not greater, need of resources.

The focus of this book is tuberculosis and its management in the United Kingdom, but as has been shown it is the cases that are brought in from less developed countries that swell the statistics and provoke panic. Therefore, its incidence in those countries is also of relevance to the discussion, and for tuberculosis to be brought under control in less developed countries, the DOT strategy must be abandoned.

PART THREE

Epidemiology

CHAPTER 7

Decline of Tuberculosis in the UK 1800–2005

The 18th century agricultural revolution led, among other things, to a decline in fatalities from tuberculosis. Parish Registers provide us with a fairly accurate record of the trend, showing a decline of one per cent annually over the ensuing century. What we are not certain about is whether people with tuberculosis who lived longer were infectious for longer periods. This would mean an increase in prevalence of tuberculosis. Increased resistance to disease owing to improved nutrition may also have mitigated the increased prevalence of the disease. Improved transportation meant equitable distribution of food and the disappearance of seasonal starvation and hunger during adverse weather conditions and following bad harvests. The annual tuberculosis mortality rate in children aged from nought to four years in the 1850s in England was 600 per 100,000 children. It was halved by the end of that century.

We may assume that better health would have an impact on tuberculosis, but we are uncertain as to how much. We know from experience in less developed countries that steadily increasing standards of nutrition have had little impact unless accompanied by reduced birth rates. No country has shown a decline in tuberculosis without such a parallel decline in its births.

The industrial revolution improved the economic condition of the population but at a huge cost as regards living conditions. Tuberculosis was rife until late in the 19th century, when rates began to fall, a trend that has continued without interruption. There was little improvement in living and social conditions but a trend, never to be reversed, of decline in birth rates in all classes of the population.

As seen, tuberculosis spreads from person to person but it is a difficult disease to catch: for a person to contract tuberculosis it is necessary to spend much time in the presence of a person who has it and is coughing. This limits the number of people who are exposed to tuberculosis. Exposure is only likely to take place in family members within a household. The number of people in a household unit will reflect the number of people being infected.

It takes about eight to 12 weeks for transmission to occur from one family member to another. There is a 30 per cent chance for a family member to contract tuberculosis infection. It is less than five per cent in the rest of the population. The smaller the family, the less opportunity there is for tuberculosis to be transmitted. Birth rates have dramatically decreased in the past half-century, from 2.9 children per family to an average of 1.8. Less than a third of households have dependent children.

By the middle of the 20th century, it was possible to predict an irreversible downward trend in tuberculosis cases in the United Kingdom, resulting from the cumulative effect of the decline spread over a century because of a continuous lowering of birth rates. The greatest decline took place before curative treatment became available in the second half of the century. Tuberculosis infection was being halved every 10 to 15 years before the availability of treatment.

What effect did treatment have on the further decline of tuberculosis in addition to that due to the diminishing birth rate? Did it make much difference? It is difficult to tell. No doubt treatment removed suffering and pain, but did it significantly add to the decrease in the prevalence of tuberculosis?

The spectacular change in the risk of infection in the Netherlands in the last century illustrates the profound alteration in the prevalence of infection as a result of the lower birth rate. The estimated number of persons infected annually with tubercle bacilli in the Netherlands in 1910 was 11,300 per 100,000 population. It was already around 500 when treatment became available. In 1945, 60 per cent of the Dutch population was infected with tubercle bacilli. From 1945 to 1985, the proportion of persons infected with tuberculosis fell from 60 per cent to 18 per cent. The proportion of infected people is estimated to be six per cent in 2005. With present trends the disease will be eradicated by 2025.

The striking reduction in infection in the post-treatment era must be studied in the context of diminished tuberculosis in the period preceding that time and the dramatic secular trends in the demography of the United Kingdom in the last half of the 20th century. The role of treatment in reducing transmission then becomes clear and the credit given to it in the irreversible decline of tuberculosis is put into perspective – additive but not very significant.

The average annual lowering of the rate of tuberculosis in the pre-treatment era was about five per cent. It soon accelerated to 10 per cent and then 15 per cent in the post-treatment period, which continues today. The traditional treatment was confined to curing active disease. This would certainly have reduced transmission of some infection but not most of it. Besides there were other powerful secular factors at work, which would have a profound effect on the transmission of tuberculosis. The most important change, discounting the lower birth rate, was in the pattern of family structure. Not only was the birth rate further reduced, making it difficult for tuberculosis to transmit, but the nuclear family which became the norm no longer housed three generations together – grandparents, parents and children. The main source of infection – grandparents – was removed, leaving parents and children in the family unit. Since parents themselves were no longer the source of tuberculosis infection, children became free of tuberculosis. Thus without treatment, tuberculosis would have eventually self-eliminated, though perhaps taking a longer time.

It is only now that we have begun to appreciate that to stop transmission we must not only treat the disease early but also treat infection arising from it. It may not be of importance in the native-born population, where risk of transmission is very low but it is of importance in people born abroad who carry high rates of infection. Death from a curable disease and continued significant transmission in children in the United Kingdom point to treatment failure. In such circumstances, it is difficult to claim that treatment has a predominant role in the decline of tuberculosis.

The importance of treatment lies in people who were born abroad in countries with high prevalence of tuberculosis. If there were a danger of an epidemic in the United Kingdom, then it would be in this population. The native population will proceed to elimination of its tuberculosis, as is predicted, by the end of the first quarter of this century. This is inevitable; the decline has gone too far to be reversible.

China and India are contrasting studies in this respect. Both began as self-governing nations 60 years ago. Both had similar patterns of tuberculosis. Today, China, because of its one-child family policy, has a tuberculosis rate approaching that of developed countries, while India lags significantly behind, as does most of the less developed world, because of high birth rates. Treatment has made little impact in countries with high population growth rates, despite improving economic conditions and nutritional standards.

No country in the world has a low prevalence of tuberculosis unaccompanied by a low birth rate. Treatment may diminish transmission of tuberculosis in individual cases, but it is powerless to influence prevalence of tuberculosis. There is no immediate prospect of decline in tuberculosis in countries with high birth rates.

The most formidable obstacle to eradicating tuberculosis in the United Kingdom immediately is the elderly population, infected in past decades. These people continue to be the main source of tuberculosis even if the population is virtually cleared of new infection. In the Netherlands (the United Kingdom shares similar conditions) in 1973 to 1980, the average annual incidence of tuberculosis among those aged 65 to 74 years was nine per 100,000 population, and in persons aged 75 years or more, it was 17 per 100,000 population. The estimated prevalence of infection in both these groups exceeded 90 per cent of the total national infection in 1975. It may be assumed that nearly all these subjects must have been infected in their early lifetime. This generation is now passing away. In the Netherlands, as in the United Kingdom, the estimated prevalence of infection will be 0.9 per cent in the year 2025. The expected incidence of infectious tuberculosis will be less than one per million – the figure proposed for tuberculosis eradication.

But in today's climate of significant numbers of people moving around the world it is not only this sector of the population that has to be considered, as I demonstrate in the next chapter.

CHAPTER 8

Epidemics in Less Developed Countries and their Influence on Tuberculosis in the UK

Tuberculosis prevalence was high, but declining at an annual rate of five per cent, before treatment against tuberculosis became available in the United Kingdom 50 years ago.

The rates in less developed countries in contrast to the developed world have lagged behind even following availability of treatment. With a few exceptions they have instead risen, sometimes to dramatic levels never experienced in the world before. There is now a much greater disparity in rates between developed and less developed countries than ever before and the gap is widening.

The main reason for the increase in tuberculosis is the population explosion that occurred in less developed countries during the second half of the 20th century. Tuberculosis has a sensitive link to overcrowding, family size and structure. Natural decline has not proved possible because of the population increase – even though many less developed countries have achieved relative prosperity with self-supporting economies and access to health care, clean water and fresh food. China and other Asian Pacific countries that have exceptionally managed to lower their birth rates are now experiencing decline in tuberculosis even without significant input from treatment of the disease.

The experience in developed countries shows that natural decline following decrease in family size is the key to the disappearance of tuberculosis. Treatment cannot on its own, without the accompanying decline in birth rates, lead to reduction in the disease.

Because tuberculosis spreads through close contacts in families, its incidence in crowded, confined places is obvious, but another demographic factor is the tradition of three generations living together making it easier for tuberculosis to be transmitted from one generation to another. Despite the one-child family structure in China, the multi-generational pattern of households, as opposed to the nuclear structure in the West, has impeded a more rapid decline of tuberculosis in that country.

With increasing family size and lack of resources to provide treatment, the rates of tuberculosis have reached epidemic proportions in many less developed countries, especially those with civil unrest, conflict, famines and floods. For example, while prevalence of tuberculosis in India is 200 per 100,000 population, it is recorded as 1,200 to 2,000 per 100,000 population in the African Horn.

The key to the persistence of tuberculosis is exposure to it. Reduce exposure, tuberculosis declines and disappears. Tuberculosis is an infectious disease and no race is more vulnerable to it than another. Rich or poor, all are equally prone if exposed to it. Tuberculosis, when treated, is cured at the same rate whether the people suffering from it are poor or rich.

Influence on prevalence of tuberculosis infection brought into the UK by people born abroad in countries with high prevalence of the disease

The infection in the population born abroad is the predominant cause of resurgence of tuberculosis in the developed world. Global migration of people from high to low prevalence countries has resurrected tuberculosis in the developed world.

The nature of immigration to the United Kingdom changed over the past two decades. Initially, it was from just a few former British colonies with good health services and social order, and then later from other disparate countries. It was no longer an orderly process of pre-arranged arrival, but of hundreds and thousands of people – homeless, refugees and asylum seekers – milling around the developed world, arriving at the borders without notice. Some who were not successful in entering the country legitimately would do so illegally.

The new arrivals causing the increase were predominantly people from countries with disintegrating health and social services. This change of immigration pattern influenced rates of incidence of tuberculosis. Immigration from Africa, where the rates are very high, has increased in the past 20 years. The trends of tuberculosis decline were reversed in

1993 coinciding with the beginning of arrivals of large numbers of black Africans to the country.

That tuberculosis has decreased in the native-born population and the number of cases in people born abroad – a much smaller population – is much greater, absolutely and relatively, is obvious from Table 1.

The decline of tuberculosis in people born abroad once they are resident in the United Kingdom

An aspect of tuberculosis epidemiology in developed countries is that rates decrease in all segments of the population at all times in a developed country.

Table 1 Proportion of tuberculosis cases occurring in the population born the United Kingdom and those born abroad 1965–1993

Year	Population	
	UK-born (94 per cent)	Born abroad (6 per cent)
1965	83.5	16.4
1971	68.2	30.7
1978/9	57	42
1983	55	45
1988	53	47
1993 (reversal of pattern)	**44**	**56**

The decline in tuberculosis in people born abroad begins immediately after entry into the country as the intense exposure to tuberculosis infection and re-infection ceases at once. But the decline in tuberculosis in people born abroad after arrival in this country starts from a much higher plateau. Tuberculosis results from infection acquired abroad. Each case of the disease means one fewer case of infection. It is a slow process of decrease but there is no increase in infection. Most of the infection, after five years of residence, will not ever lead to disease. The decline is imperceptible but cumulative. It matters that an infection is on hold or even decreasing with time. It means outbreaks are not likely to occur despite the overwhelming presence of tuberculosis infection in people born abroad.

Recently acquired infection is the most important cause of tuberculosis in any population. Recent infection in a person born in a high prevalence country is the predominant contributor to the tuberculosis load in the United Kingdom. Five per cent of infection acquired within five years before entry results in tuberculosis, and then another five per cent of infection leads to disease over the rest of a lifetime.

Once the acquired infection is five years old, or the person from abroad has lived in the United Kingdom for five years or more, the rate of progression of infection to tuberculosis becomes similar to that in native-born people. Infection in black Africans tends to be of recent origin – hence the disproportionate contribution to tuberculosis from this source (less than one per cent of the population) in the United Kingdom.

It is not the prevalence of tuberculosis in the resident

country that is of importance in determining its incidence, but the rate of unstable infection that is imported into the country. It is erroneous to believe that people born abroad have a tendency towards tuberculosis, an inborn weakness resulting from environmental, economical, nutritional, or behavioural influences, or that some of these factors, such as deprivation, overcrowding and nutritional deficiency, continue to influence the incidence of tuberculosis after the arrival of these people in the host countries.

The incidence of tuberculosis in people born abroad on first arrival is due to the natural history of the infection in their country of origin. No social, environmental or economic explanation is needed.

The decline of tuberculosis in the people born abroad who have settled in the United Kingdom is illustrated by the example of the Indian community.

In the United Kingdom, Indians are the largest group of people born abroad. This population, compared with the native population, shows an increasing total number of cases owing to additional immigration, but declining rates reflecting the epidemiology in India. Indians bring in mostly stable infection from India, which leads to disease at the same rate as in the native-born population. In contrast, black Africans bring in unstable infection and contribute to tuberculosis in far greater numbers in proportion to their population (see Table 2).

In Table 2, the population includes Indians born abroad, and first, second and third generations born in the United

Kingdom. Rates reflect averages of intergenerational declining rates.

The pattern of decline between the first and subsequent immigrant generations is marked. The first generation has greater exposure to tuberculosis at home from parents born abroad with a greater load of infection.

The second and third generations are only exposed to parents born in the United Kingdom but may because of family structure become exposed to grandparents, uncles and aunts born abroad. In practice such increased exposure to tuberculosis is a passing trend and not important epidemiologically. The rates of tuberculosis are not much different from those of any other population group born in the United Kingdom.

The continuous decline has important implications for the management of tuberculosis in people born abroad: no additional steps are necessary. They pose no major

Table 2 Trends in annual notification rates per 100,000 Indian population in the United Kingdom

1978/79		1983		1988	
Population (000)	Rate per 100,000	Population (000)	Rate per 100,000	Population (000)	Rate per 100,000
43,320	9.4	42,994	6.9	43,938	4.7

epidemiological risk to themselves or others. Taking into account the rapid natural decline in rates once they are resident in the country, a holding policy with medical treatment alone suffices: cases are treated as they arise and close contacts investigated and treated for new infection.

Influence on spread (transmission) of tuberculosis in the United Kingdom with arrival of people born abroad in high tuberculosis countries

Has tuberculosis returned because of immigration from the less developed world with very high tuberculosis rates?

It has returned if the previously uninfected native-born population increasingly begins to contract infection and the rate of infection begins to increase in this population – if the native population has succumbed to the disease and the infection has now taken hold of the segment of the population previously unaffected. Alternatively, immigrants bring in the infection and increase the number of cases of tuberculosis, but have no influence on tuberculosis in the native-born population.

Tuberculosis prevalence in the population born abroad has an overall impact on tuberculosis *numbers* in the United Kingdom, but it has no impact on the risk of infection in the native-born population. The native-born population does not suffer from increased tuberculosis due to high rates in the population born abroad, even when there is an increase in the total number of cases of tuberculosis in the country. There is no change in the trend in the inevitable decline in tuberculosis in the native-born population in the United Kingdom, but the population base (denominator) has changed and overall tuberculosis numbers have risen dramatically.

Tuberculosis does not spread from people born abroad to the population born in the United Kingdom. The greater the number of people born in a country with high prevalence of tuberculosis infection, the higher the prevalence in the host country – adding to the number of cases reported. The increase in number of cases is not due to an increased spread but is a function of the continuing increase in the number of new arrivals over time. The increased number of cases does not contribute to increased rates. These, as suggested above, always show downward trends.

Tuberculosis in the native-born population, for which predictions of eradication were made 50 years ago, is still on course and is on the path to elimination within the next three decades. The trends in the native-born population have never changed. Rates are already as low as one per 100,000 population in infants and children. Tuberculosis is now generally confined to older people, arising from old infection acquired decades earlier.

If there were no further increase in the number of people arriving in this country from high prevalence countries, tuberculosis would eventually decline and disappear from all sections of the population.

CHAPTER 9

Molecular DNA Evidence for Source of Infection in Immigrants in Israel and Denmark

The use of DNA fingerprinting to distinguish epidemiologically related and unrelated strains of *M. tuberculosis* confirms that tuberculosis in immigrants is linked to infection in the country of their origin. Tuberculosis prevalence varies enormously in the less developed world but it is always much higher, even at its lowest rates, than that in the developed world.

DNA studies show that the source of infection lies in the country of origin. Even clusters of cases (outbreaks), which suggest recent transmission but are chance occurrences, can be traced back to infection acquired abroad. Israel accepts proportionately more immigrants than any other country in the world and Denmark has an immigration pattern similar to the United Kingdom. DNA studies to establish the source of infection in these two countries are described below.

Israel

The incidence of tuberculosis in the native-born population

is four cases per 100,000. The tuberculosis rates for recent immigrants from the former Soviet Union countries (38 to 172 per 100,000 population) and Ethiopia (500 to 2,000 per 100,000 population) are much higher. From 1990 to 1996, Israel absorbed more than 750,000 immigrants, one seventh of the whole population.

Results of molecular epidemiology show that each infected immigrant imports the tubercle bacillus from his or her country of birth and that the disease is reactivated in the country of domicile, often soon after arrival. No cross-infection occurs between the new immigrants themselves or the local population. Tuberculosis among the immigrants is mainly from reactivation of latent infection.

Denmark

Since 1986, the number of tuberculosis patients reported in Denmark has increased by 91 per cent. The incidence has remained stable in the native-born population. The increase is explained by immigration from countries with a high prevalence of the disease. The Somalis in Denmark have a prevalence of 2,000 per 100,000 population, which is among the highest ever reported in the world (100 per cent of all adults and 25 per cent of all children are tuberculin test positive on arrival). Eighty per cent of all new cases develop within two years of arrival.

Two thirds of all tuberculosis cases reported in Denmark are in immigrants and half are from Somalia. Molecular epidemiology showed that 55.2 per cent of Somalis shared identical DNA fingerprint patterns; 74.9 per cent of these were most likely infected before their arrival in Denmark, 23.3 per cent were most likely infected in Denmark by other Somalis. In the same period, only 0.9 per cent of all Danish tuberculosis patients were most likely infected by Somalis. *M. tuberculosis* transmission among Somalis in Denmark is limited, and transmission between Somalis and Danes is nearly non-existent.

This confirms the view that any increase in prevalence of cases in a host country is confined to the population bringing the disease in.

CHAPTER 10

Influence of Medical Treatment on Tuberculosis in the USA: Epidemic Resurgence to Elimination

In a developed country, resurgence of tuberculosis occurs for two reasons. It is an epidemic if it results from rapid person-to-person transmission on a large scale. Non-epidemic resurgence, on the other hand, results from mass migration of infected persons from countries with high rates of tuberculosis. The USA not only suffers from non-epidemic tuberculosis resurgence like other developed countries but has also experienced an epidemic unlike that seen in any other developed country in modern times.

Tuberculosis epidemic USA 1986–1992

The United States suffered the worst ever epidemic of tuberculosis in modern times in the developed world during the period between 1986 and 1992. The resurgence of tuberculosis was marked by several years of increasing case counts followed by a sudden, steeper rise for several years in the mid-1980s. Tuberculosis was used metaphorically in Victorian English literature to describe aesthetic beauty, pale, delicate, passive and gracefully fading away to death, but the metaphor for the United States epidemic was an unforgiving, free market economy that took no hostage, offered no shelter for the poor, sick and downtrodden – the margins of its society.

The resurgence in numbers of tuberculosis cases in the developed world in recent times is now well documented. It is due to the increase in the number of already infected immigrants from countries with high tuberculosis rates. The role of active transmission from person to person in the developed world, even in recent arrivals, is small compared with the total pool of infection in the community. The United States, in contrast, suffered from an epidemic with intense active transmission from one person to another, reversing the continuing downward progression of the disease.

In the United States during the period 1953 to 1985 the number of tuberculosis cases dropped from 84,304 to 22,201 notifications (74 per cent), an average annual decline of six per cent. The United States stopped public funding of treatment of tuberculosis under the impression, though it proved to be false, that it was no longer necessary. However, what was hidden by the decline in number of cases were pockets of high tuberculosis infection in marginalised segments of the population – the urban poor, destitute and homeless – who were without treatment. New York was the epicentre of the epidemic, and a quarter of the population who developed tuberculosis had no access to treatment. The result was the uncontrolled spread of the disease.

The reason for the resurgence in the United States was the withdrawal of free tuberculosis treatment. Coincidental outbreaks of HIV/AIDS and intravenous drug abuse had a multiplier effect on transmission of tuberculosis from one person to another. The force of explosion of tuberculosis was further intensified by the development of resistance to anti-tuberculosis drugs, when availability of free medical treatment was already minimal and inadequate. It made the epidemic even more complex and difficult to deal with.

Unlike the situation in other developed countries, it was the native-born population who bore the brunt of the intense transmission of tuberculosis infection – the deprived and homeless people in prisons and shelters in the United States. The ground was laid for the invisible tuberculosis infection epidemic to become overt when the government unwittingly stepped into the lull before the storm and stopped public expenditure on treatment.

In 1985, the tuberculosis rates decreased by only one tenth of one per cent; this was followed by an increase, for the first time in the 20th century, of 1.1 per cent over the 1985 rates during 1986. It was to reach a peak average annual increase of five per cent in 1992 with 26,673 cases. The dramatic increase is reflected in the numbers – 70,000 cases more than anticipated between 1985 and 1993. From 1985 through to 1992, the tuberculosis epidemic in the United States resulted in an increase in the number of cases in children – a measure of active (person to person) transmission.

Race differences in access to health services provided a vivid explanation for the different rates of tuberculosis in different segments of the American population. The definition of native-born people with universal low rates of tuberculosis did not hold true in the United States. The incidence of tuberculosis in the United States-born population in 1997 was high in the "natives" (13.4 per cent), blacks (20.5 per cent), and Hispanics (14.4 per cent), in clear contrast to the rate in non-Hispanic whites (2.5 per cent).

A renewed emphasis on tuberculosis control in the 1990s resulted in a rapid, substantial decline in the spread of the disease from person to person from within the country and from causes other than immigration to the United States.

The interrupted decline began again in 1993, the reported incidence of tuberculosis being 9.8 cases per 100,000 population representing a 5.2 per cent decrease from the 1992 rate. This decline was still 14 per cent greater than the 1985 rate. In 1994, the number of cases decreased again by 3.7 per cent, as compared with 1993. By 1998, the caseload was 18,361 (a case rate of 6.8 per 100,000 population), a decline of 31 per cent over the previous five years. From 1992 until 2002, the total number of tuberculosis cases decreased by five to seven per cent annually. The year 2005 marked the 13th year of decline in the total number of tuberculosis cases reported in the United States following the peak of the epidemic a decade earlier.

Interim progress towards elimination of tuberculosis 2002

The interim stage marks epidemiological cessation of transmission of tuberculosis in the native-born population, predominance of tuberculosis in foreign-born people and decline of incidence in all segments of the population, born in the United States or abroad.

A total of 15,078 tuberculosis cases were reported in 2002, representing a 5.7 per cent decline from 2001 and a 43.5 per cent decline from the 1992 peak of the epidemic. It was the lowest recorded tuberculosis rate in the United States since reporting began in 1953.

The renewed decline since 1992 has taken place in all age groups, racial/ethnic populations, and regions of the United States. Despite this progress, the 2002 rate of 5.2 cases per 100,000 population remained higher than the 2000 interim goal of 3.5, set as part of the national strategic plan for tuberculosis elimination (less than one case per 1,000,000 by 2010).

Overall national decline in tuberculosis incidence masks substantial disparities between rates in the three segments of the population: US-born white persons, foreign-born persons and US-born non-Hispanic blacks. The latter two segments of the population now account for three quarters of tuberculosis cases.

Further progress towards tuberculosis elimination in the United States will depend on (1) specific programmes that provide services to foreign-born persons with tuberculosis infection, and (2) intensified tuberculosis control efforts that address higher tuberculosis rates in the US-born non-Hispanic black population.

During 1992 to 2002, case rates declined in all but three states. Five states (California, Florida, Illinois, New York and Texas) accounted for 52.5 per cent of cases and 68.3 per cent of the overall decrease in the number of cases; case rates in these states declined on average by approximately 50 per cent. The proportion of patients with multi-drug-resistant tuberculosis (i.e. resistance to at least two anti-tuberculosis drugs) decreased from 486 (2.7 per cent) in 1993 to 138 (1.3 per cent) of 10,601 cases in 2002.

Rates declined in both the US-born and the foreign-born population between 1992 and 2002. However, the decline was substantially less among the foreign-born population and the ratio of foreign-born to US-born rates doubled, from 4.2 in 1992 to 8.4 in 2002. In 2002, for the first time, tuberculosis cases among foreign-born persons accounted for the majority (51.0 per cent) of tuberculosis cases in the United States. The number of states with more than 50 per cent of cases among foreign-born persons increased from four in 1992 to 22 in 2002. In seven states, approximately 70 per cent of cases were among foreign-born persons. As in 1992, the most common birth countries for foreign-born persons with tuberculosis in 2002 were Mexico (24.8 per cent), the Philippines (11.3 per cent), Vietnam (8.6 per cent), India (7.6 per cent), China (4.5 per cent), Haiti (3.4 per cent), and South Korea (2.7 per cent).

Despite a 68.4 per cent decline in rates from 1992, US-born non-Hispanic blacks in 2002 continued to have the highest tuberculosis rate of any US-born racial/ethnic population or indeed any foreign-born population; they had 46.7 per cent of tuberculosis cases in US-born persons and approximately one quarter of all cases.

Of US-born racial/ethnic populations, rates among non-

Hispanic blacks were 7.5 times and 2.1 times higher than those among non-Hispanic whites and Hispanics, respectively. The latter two US-born groups account for the majority of tuberculosis cases. Since 1992, when tuberculosis cases in the US peaked after seven years of increasing rates, there has been a decline by on average five per cent per year. The strengthened tuberculosis control efforts that have been effective in reversing increases in rates among US-born persons have had far less effect on rates among foreign-born persons.

CHAPTER 11

Tuberculosis in the UK 1993–2005

Tuberculosis rates have risen for at least the last consecutive 15 years. The increase in 2002 was four per cent above the rate in 2001 (see Table 3). More cases were reported in people born abroad than in native-born for the first time in 1993.

The main difference in the epidemiology of tuberculosis between the United Kingdom and the United States in the period 1985 to 1995 is the proportion of cases transmitted from person to person as a result of the epidemic of tuberculosis in the United States.

In the United Kingdom, as we have seen, the non-epidemic resurgence is due to the arrival of persons from countries with high rates of tuberculosis and the increase in number of cases is because of the progress of imported infection to overt disease in the country. There was little transmission of tuberculosis to contribute to the upsurge itself, in contrast to significant transmission from person to person within the USA. Indeed, during this period, there has been a continuous decline of active transmission in the face of increasing numbers of cases in all groups of the population in the United Kingdom.

In 2002, 6,907 tuberculosis cases were reported. This was an increase of 3.7 per cent over 2001. Sixty-three per cent of

Table 3 Number of tuberculosis case reports in England and Wales

Year	Number of cases	Percentage change in rate
1988	4,659	7.5
1993	**5,104**	**7.5**
1998	5,658	10.0
1999	5,704	0.0
2000	6,271	10.0
2001	6,597	5.0
2002	6,907	3.7

persons with tuberculosis were born abroad (four per cent of the total population), representing an average rate of 73.0 per 100,000 population compared with a prevalence of less than 4.3 per cent in those born in the United Kingdom (94 per cent of the population). The prevalence was 211 per 100,000 in black Africans, 145 in Pakistanis, and 104 in Indians.

The largest proportion of cases was reported in the London region (41 per cent, incidence 38 per 100,000 population) followed by the West Midlands (11 per cent, incidence 13.7 per 100,000 population) – the two regions with the highest proportion of people born abroad. In areas with a limited immigrant population, the incidence by region was Eastern 6.1 per cent, South East 5.9 per cent, and South West 4.4 per cent.

Tuberculosis has a strong urban association, as this is where most of the people born abroad reside. London accounts for the highest proportion of all cases (43 per cent) with the highest rate of tuberculosis (43 cases per 100,000 population). Of the total population of people born abroad, 30 per cent live in London.

Tuberculosis is cured with treatment. The number of deaths during the year 2001 was 427, eight per cent of the notifications of tuberculosis. Deaths reflect treatment failure. Prompt diagnosis and treatment halt transmission. Preventing transmission is the gold standard for effective control of the disease. Treatment of recently acquired infection, when transmission does take place, and preventive treatment of all contacts of tuberculosis under the age of five years will end transmission. Transmission is not inevitable. It is within the bounds of treatment.

It has been shown here that the cause of the resurgence of tuberculosis in the United Kingdom lies in people born abroad. Transmission of infection, on the other hand, reflects failure of control in the United Kingdom. One is not avoidable, the other is. Existing infection in the native-born population, with which we are historically bound, and increased migration of people born abroad should be unlinked from the inevitable incidence of the disease or at least that part of it associated with transmission owing to failure of treatment in the United Kingdom.

CHAPTER 12

Factors Determining Risk of Tuberculosis Infection in the UK

Intensity of infection in a population predicts the level of disease in a population. It is not practically possible to measure the incidence of infection in people born in the United Kingdom. The annual risk of infection with tubercle bacilli is derived from results of tuberculin test surveys in large numbers of persons. Several tuberculin test surveys are required, at intervals, at different ages, each survey taking a sample of non-BCG-vaccinated subjects of the same age. A representative sample of same age non-BCG persons is not possible as universal BCG vaccination is offered to all children in the country.

BCG was never introduced in Holland. As the pattern of tuberculosis in Holland is similar to that of other developed countries, it serves as a typical illustration for trends in tuberculosis risk in developed countries (see Table 4).

There is no linear relationship between the risk of infection and the incidence of tuberculosis. Annual risk of tuberculosis infection has declined from 0.6 per cent in the 1950s to 0.01 per cent 50 years later, but the disease has lagged behind and has not followed the risk pattern. The reason is that the majority of cases in the native-born population occur in adults who acquired their infection decades earlier. This is therefore not reflected in current risk of developing infection.

Trends in risk of infection, even where changes shown seem minimal, are of importance in shaping the course of tuberculosis. When regular decrease, however small, is achieved, an accelerating effect sets in with tremendous force. Even with the slightest continuous decrease, every successive birth year will set in a pattern of irreversible decreasing risk of infection.

A portion of older people who had experienced the highest risk of infection during their childhood, adolescence and young adulthood is removed by death each year, adding further to the decline in the risk of disease. Once old infection has died out, the levels of infection currently acquired will be sufficiently low for tuberculosis to self-eliminate within a short period of time.

With an annual decline in infection of 10 per cent since treatment became available 50 years ago, the risk of infection in the native-born population has reduced to a small

Table 4 Prevalence of tuberculosis in 10-year cohorts in Holland

Year of birth	Prevalence in 1985 (%)
1905	90.0
1915	74.0
1925	49.0
1935	24.0
1945	7.5
1955	2.4
1965	0.07
1985	0.012

percentage. The effect is compounded in successive years. Generations with successively decreasing levels of infection are replacing older generations with higher rates of infection.

The risk of infection at the beginning of the century was so large that no person could escape it before reaching young adulthood. In the developed world, a risk of infection of around 30 per cent is now reduced to between 0.1 and 0.01 per cent.

The qualitative difference in tuberculosis in low and high prevalence countries is important. Transmission in the former is incrementally reduced with time as fewer opportunities for infection occur, while it remains the same or even increases in the latter depending on the intensity of the infection.

It is not possible to define precisely the period of the primary tuberculosis phase, but it ends when the immune process starts to contain the infection. In the beginning, the containment is fragile; breakdown is common.

Tuberculosis enters the secondary, stable phase five years after the infection is first acquired. Less than 0.01 per cent infection leads to disease annually. Tuberculosis is best understood as the primary phase lasting five years and the secondary phase lasting the rest of the lifetime. In high intensity infection countries, frequent re-infection means that an infected person remains perpetually in the primary phase and continues to carry highly unstable infection, with a greatly enhanced chance of progressing to active disease.

The immune process does not have the ability to kill all the tubercle bacilli. The bacilli are viable but dormant, contained within a fragile cocoon. Stability the live but dormant tubercle bacilli focus is continuously compromised owing to the fragile nature of the primary phase. The resolution of the primary phase results in a highly stable secondary phase, but still containing viable tubercle bacilli.

The acquired immunity inhibits multiplication of the tuberculosis bacteria, but not their destruction. The bacteria are held in check in dormant foci but they are capable of dividing again (endogenous reactivation) by mechanisms that are as yet poorly understood. Endogenous reactivation is independent of the risk of infection.

Endogenous flare-up of a dormant infection is the most common cause of adult tuberculosis in the native-born population in a low risk country, as is demonstrated by the low prevalence of the disease in children where an exogenous source (external infection) would be necessary to cause infection.

As the risk declines, the majority of tuberculosis cases are due to endogenous exacerbation. Where the risk is still high, exogenous infection remains high and tuberculosis is found at all ages, especially in childhood.

In countries with high rates, continuous exposure to tuberculosis results in unstable infection. When people with unstable infection arrive in the United Kingdom, a proportion of the unstable infection leads to tuberculosis within a short period. It is this tuberculosis which is responsible for the increasing incidence.

In countries with low rates of tuberculosis, re-infection is uncommon. People born in countries with intermediate, but stable, infection contribute to rates at a much slower pace, spread over decades, and make a lower overall contribution to the tuberculosis load. India is an example.

The most recent arrivals have higher rates of tuberculosis than those who have lived here longer. The notification of tuberculosis in arrivals from Pakistan was 77 times greater than for Pakistanis who had been resident in the UK for 10 years. Notifications in immigrants from India, within two years of their arrival in England, showed a rate 63 times greater than for those who had been resident for five years.

We know that 50 per cent of tuberculosis results from recent contacts of a case of tuberculosis. Recent immigrants are at highest risk, sometimes several hundred-fold higher, as they are likely to import recent, unstable infection from their country of origin. But labelling and investigating with a view to reducing levels of risk to different groups of the population produces poor results in controlling tuberculosis. Attaching level of risk to population segments would be a bureaucratic nightmare without benefit.

Summary of specific risk factors for tuberculosis in the native-born population

Close contacts

Close contacts of people with tuberculosis are at the highest risk of developing infection. Close contacts are family members and intimate friends.

Recent infection

Persons who have recently acquired infection are at the highest risk of developing the disease. The risk of tuberculosis disease in recent tuberculosis-infected contacts is 15 times greater as compared with the risk for people with no known contact. Fifty per cent of tuberculosis results from recent contacts of a case of infectious tuberculosis in a short period of time.

Age

Tuberculosis is most common in old age. Elderly people were exposed to high levels of infection as children and young people. The elderly are more likely to develop tuberculosis because they carry a high load of the infection. Of all cases reported in 2002, the highest rates were in people of 50 years of age and older. Tuberculosis case rates were 25+ per 100,000 population in people aged 80 years and over.

Reduced immunity

Reduced immunity may result in people suffering from HIV/AIDS, malnutrition, alcoholism, drug addiction and chronic diseases. Reduced immunity is not an important factor for tuberculosis.

PART FOUR

Policy for the Control of Tuberculosis

CHAPTER 13

Formulating a Hypothesis for Tuberculosis Taking into Account Demographic, Epidemiological and Pathological Factors

Uncertainty surrounds tuberculosis. I propose a hypothesis for readers to accept or reject.

The hypothesis proposes that tuberculosis is in an inevitable decline in the United Kingdom. Its demise will be hastened by early curative treatment and retarded by policies that postpone or inhibit this.

A unified theory is described here to satisfy the criteria for the hypothesis, which draws together the strands that influence the natural history of tuberculosis in the United Kingdom. The factors considered in this book are demographic, epidemiological and pathological, and the discussion below brings together the elements of the whole picture, some of which have been touched on earlier.

Demographic factors

Tuberculosis is a complex disease. Demographic patterns and environmental interactions are key to its transmission. These impinge in an incremental way on the natural history of the disease to produce negative or positive additive change over time.

In developed countries, tuberculosis fails to transmit itself, which will after a predictable period lead to its self-elimination, whereas in less developed countries, spread is such that epidemics of tuberculosis are continually being experienced.

The most intense exposure to tuberculosis occurs in people who share a household. Children are exposed to their parents and older siblings in the nuclear family structure that is a norm in developed countries. Exposure to grandparents, who are much more likely to carry infection from the past, is not at a level which will result in successful exposure to tuberculosis in children.

The birth rate is less than two children per nuclear family. The number of children exposed is decreased, even if the probability of tuberculosis occurring in an adult remains unchanged. The sleeping arrangements, with children assigned their own bedrooms, further reduce the chance of successful exposure to tuberculosis.

While transmission of tuberculosis within a household is the most important factor in the spread of disease, its failure to do so in a typical family means that it is unable to perpetuate and must therefore eliminate itself in time.

In less developed countries, where birth rates are high, the population has increased exponentially, and three or even four generations may live together in crowded conditions, sharing limited space with each other. Exposure to infection is intense and so is the spread of tuberculosis.

We have seen that the most important causal factor for tuberculosis in developed countries is the country of birth. Two thirds of all cases of tuberculosis will be found in people born in less developed countries. Such people, while contributing massively to the tuberculosis load, constitute no more than five to 10 percent of the total population.

An understanding of the population base (denominator) is essential for understanding tuberculosis. The place of birth, either in a less developed country or in a developed one, the two-nation concept, is the only factor that drives the epidemiology of tuberculosis in a developed country.

The average case rate of tuberculosis in a population born in a developed country is under four per 100,000 population. In populations born in less developed countries, the case rates vary, from over 100 to 2,000 per 100,000 population.

There will be intermediate rates in some countries. Reference is only made to developed and developing countries. These are the ones that matter epidemiologically. Rates are approximate and indicative, suggesting trends. Accurate rates are not possible to obtain, and are not relevant in discussing the natural history of tuberculosis in the modern world.

Race and ethnic population denominators confound the epidemiology. Moslem children born in a developed country belong to a segment of the population with a caseload of one to two per 100,000 population. Moslem children born in African Horn countries belong to a population group with a tuberculosis case rate of 1,000 per 100,000 population. An average case rate of tuberculosis in the Moslem population in a developed country has no meaning, epidemiologically or statistically.

Within the same family, a Moslem child born in the United Kingdom and a sibling born in an African Horn country will belong to two groups with vastly different rates of tuberculosis. These never intertwine.

Tuberculosis rates in segments of population by race and ethnicity in the United Kingdom give an unfortunate impression that tuberculosis has a propensity in certain races because of genetic, gender or socio-economic conditions. This is not true in the United Kingdom. Only the country of birth is relevant to the epidemiology of tuberculosis.

The rates in the immigrant generations born in the United Kingdom may be higher than the rates in the native-born population as there is proportionately greater exposure to infection from parents born abroad who have high rates of infection. But such differences are not significant epidemiologically. It is safe to assume for practical purposes that all children born in the United Kingdom have the same rates of tuberculosis.

Exposure to tuberculosis infection and its transmission are the sole deciding factors in contracting the disease irrespective of racial or ethnic origin. This depends on the country of birth. The country of birth leaves an irredeemable imprint, as infection once acquired after birth remains for life. Race or ethnic experience reflects geographical origin. It is more pertinent to describe present and past exposure to tuberculosis in the population.

It is important to avoid loosely using terms such as race, ethnicity, immigrants, new arrivals, illegal entrants, overseas students, asylum seekers or refugees to suggest populations with different rates of tuberculosis. It may be occasionally true but not always. Refugees from the former Yugoslavia or east European countries have low levels of tuberculosis. In a tuberculin skin test survey in these populations, thousands of tests produced not a single case of active disease. Only country of birth decides the case rate for tuberculosis. Not political status of new arrivals.

The term "native-born" describes people whose ancestry lies in developed countries. I use the term "white" sparingly. It also has the same strength of meaning. One is either born in a developed country or in a less developed one. The term "natives" in the United States has different connotations. Readers should keep this in mind.

A feature of the native-born population is that it has never been exposed to a higher risk of tuberculosis than that shared by the whole segment of that population. A feature of such population is the decline in prevalence of tuberculosis over the past 50 years of no less than 10 per cent annually.

The native-born population (94 per cent) in the United Kingdom shares a continuous, uninterrupted decline of tuberculosis, uninfluenced by any change in the rates of tuberculosis in the population born abroad. All economically advanced countries share the same rates. Currently it is less than four per 100,000 population. It suggests powerful secular trends. Treatment plays an important but essentially supportive role. The purpose of treatment is mainly to remove suffering and pain in patients and to sustain the secular trend. The decline in rates is irreversible. Elimination of tuberculosis in people born in the United Kingdom will result in about three decades at the present rate of decline.

It is erroneous to average rates of tuberculosis in an ethnic or racial segment of the population, as such a group will have people born in less developed countries and those born locally in a developed country. For example, an Indian born abroad will share a tuberculosis caseload of about 150 per 100,000 population and to average this with a rate in locally-born Indians, about four cases per 100,000 population[1], will produce a value suggesting dramatic declining rates in those born abroad and rising rates in those born locally, which is the opposite to the picture of tuberculosis.

Similarly, to average tuberculosis case rates in 94 per cent of the population born in the United Kingdom (four per 100,000 population) and six per cent of the population born in less developed countries (100+ per 100,000 population) and come to an absurd number such as 12 cases per 100,000 population is not comparing like with like and has no statistical meaning. It will suggest an increasing tuberculosis rate in a population where it is decreasing.

Epidemiological factors

The number of new cases in a year describes the incidence in

---

1. The term "100,000 population" refers to the same population in the denominator as in the numerator and not always to the population of the country as a whole.

that year. This is the most useful piece of information about tuberculosis. It must describe rates based on country of birth in a developed or less developed country. The rates within the same population will vary enormously within different age groups. Age can also be used to further define the population base (denominator).

Prevalence is the total number of cases at any one time. It can only be estimated as there is no practical means to determine it. The word prevalence is used in this book to describe the general picture of tuberculosis in a country.

Pathological factors

Tuberculosis results either from transmission from a person with disease to a person without it (exogenous) or from reactivation of a person's own dormant infection (endogenous). It is not possible to distinguish clinically between the two but epidemiological information may provide a clue. The distinction in type of tuberculosis plays no part in the clinical management of the disease but it matters a great deal epidemiologically. If the disease is transmitted, tuberculosis is increased with new cases; if it is reactivated, no increase has taken place, and indeed there is one fewer case of tuberculosis infection. It tells us whether tuberculosis control is effective or not. It is if no transmission takes place, irrespective of the number of cases arising from reactivation of dormant infection.

Tuberculosis in adults is likely to be reactivated in both the native-born population and those born abroad. For children and young people born in the United Kingdom, it is safe to assume it to be new and transmitted. In children born abroad, it may be either reactivated or transmitted. A source must be looked for in all cases of tuberculosis in children. New (transmitted) disease is an indicator of failure in diagnosis and treatment of the index case of tuberculosis.

It is important to understand the difference between the terms infection and disease. The reference to tuberculosis without qualification, for example tuberculosis infection, is active disease, based on clinical and/or bacteriological and/or radiological evidence and/or a positive tuberculin skin test.

Infection is the key to understanding the epidemiology of tuberculosis. It is the stage where tubercle bacilli have successfully invaded and established themselves in the body. An infected person does not have the disease and cannot transmit the infection to others. Approximately one third to half of the world's population in less developed countries is infected with tuberculosis, but only a small minority will go on to develop the disease.

There are no symptoms at this stage and the infected person is not aware of his or her infection. Not all infection leads to tuberculosis. Only 10 per cent will ever do so over a lifetime. Infection is most likely to lead to tuberculosis in the early stages before the body has the opportunity to develop immunity against the infection. Infection is not infectious.

In the latter stages of the infection, when immunity is developed, tubercle bacilli stop multiplying and become dormant. Immunity is partial and not sufficient to destroy the tubercle bacilli and rid the body of them. Infection is manifested by a positive tuberculin skin test reaction without clinical symptoms and signs, bacteriological evidence or radiological abnormalities. It can lead to disease at any time during the course of a lifetime. But most infected people will die of some other cause.

Anti-tuberculosis treatment will cure infection. It is often described as preventive treatment. The treatment of tuberculosis infection prevents progression to active disease.

The tuberculosis elimination phase is achieved when the incidence of all forms of active tuberculosis falls below one per million population per year. The United States has a dedicated programme for elimination of tuberculosis in people born in the country.

The tuberculin skin test is a means to determine infection with tuberculosis. It does not differentiate natural from BCG-induced reaction. It is an unreliable test if people have previously had BCG. Its value is undermined in a person who has previously received BCG vaccination. There are also significant issues around the test's sensitivity and specificity, and hence predictive value as a tool for screening of symptomatic people. These statistical measures indicate its unreliability for screening of infection.

Readers are now equipped to examine the hypothesis, the evidence and the arguments, which are presented in the rest of the book.

CHAPTER 14

Sensitivity Distorts Tuberculosis Policy in the UK

Free enquiry transforms human understanding of the matter in hand. It reveals how things are on the basis of evidence instead of authority and hearsay. The right to know is not unfettered. Free enquiry is regulated in a democracy to preserve our other esteemed values or to take account of the way others might react to them. The asking of provocative questions to determine conclusions may be unwelcome to interest groups. People may practise self-censorship or they may find it easier to prevent moral outrage by parroting established orthodoxy, even when their enquiries point in an opposite direction.

Enquiry into tuberculosis is a subject that is off-limits. It is prohibited in the interest of racial harmony. Immigrants are responsible for the increase in the number of cases of tuberculosis in the United Kingdom. They have reversed the declining trends. To make matters worse, less than one per cent of the immigrant population is responsible for the dramatic increase in tuberculosis in recent years. Finger pointing is unacceptable.

Exploring the differences in tuberculosis epidemiology is in the area of politically correct forbidden knowledge. Yet if such differences were correct, understanding them would prove important in providing relief to the affected population itself from disease. This opportunity is unfortunately denied them, in the name of racial harmony.

We have been here before. Readers will remember the shrill sloganeering that we were all susceptible to AIDS, when over 95 per cent of the population had no reason to be at risk of contracting the disease.

It is unfortunately the case that the arrival of black Africans, a small proportion of the people from developing countries, since the mid-1990s, is responsible for the dramatic increase in the number of cases of tuberculosis. Only in areas of London and Birmingham where black Africans have settled is the problem encountered; other areas have not experienced this rise in the disease.

There is little doubt that there will be a hostile response to this statement, not because it is incorrect but because it will be crashing into a forbidden barrier. The message will be seen as unacceptable and irresponsible. It should not have brought the subject into the open in the interest of the greater good of racial harmony.

I accept that society has a right to place limits on what and how scientific information is made available, but I know from long experience of practising medicine among immigrants that those who suffer from tuberculosis welcome openness. Even more, they are eager to give information to protect family and friends from contracting the disease. The fear of stigma attached to tuberculosis is in the mind of the politically correct people and not those who suffer from it.

The United Kingdom Department of Health in "Stopping Tuberculosis: An Action Plan (2004)" offers the following hypothesis:

"Tuberculosis is a serious disease and has increased by 25 per cent over the last 10 years and is still rising. Thirteen cases in every 100,000 people were newly diagnosed for tuberculosis in England in the year 2002."

The hypothesis is a myth. No explanation is offered as to how these numbers were arrived at and therefore we cannot examine their veracity. A true hypothesis opens the mind to thought, to comparison, to doubt and to the contrariness of truth. A myth is a frozen hypothesis endlessly repeating slogans and declarations to justify the mythical truth without letting the truth itself receive a hearing. Entry of "Tuberculosis USA" in a web search engine produces the most detailed information on the disease in that country. Not so for a similar request for this country. Indeed, the action plan wistfully quotes the example of the United States, which with its clear plan turned the tide from high levels of tuberculosis to low ones within a decade.

Truth has been indeed the casualty in the manipulation of information where problems of tuberculosis are secondary to political propaganda and spin.

The policy of the United States is:

"Progress toward tuberculosis elimination in the United States will depend on (1) specific programmes that provide services to foreign-born persons with tuberculosis infection, and (2) intensified tuberculosis control efforts that address higher tuberculosis rates in the US-born black population."

The London Assembly Health Committee report "Tuberculosis in London 2003" goes further than the UK government in obfuscating the reality:

"Tuberculosis is, and always has been, disease engendered by poverty. Social and economic deprivation, particularly bad housing, is a breeding ground for tuberculosis as it has a major impact on both the transmission of the disease and the effectiveness of treatment. People most at risk are usually those with the most limited access to primary care. The disease is spread unevenly across the capital; hitting those areas where deprivation is high."

The report ignores the fact that only in areas where black Africans reside are problems of tuberculosis manifested. Other areas of London, equally if not more deprived, which do not have black Africans, suffer no such rise of the disease.

Tuberculosis is an infectious disease that responds fully to treatment. Even after treatment, the rich will stay rich and the poor, poor. That was the clear United States policy, which both the Government and London Assembly admire so much but fail to practice.

The hypothesis which I propose and which I examine in this book is as follows:

Since records of infectious disease began in the 19th century, tuberculosis has been in decline in the developed world. The current rate of decline is around 15 per cent. Tuberculosis will be eliminated in people born in the United Kingdom (94 per cent of the population) towards the end of the first quarter of this century.

Increase in the incidence of tuberculosis results when there is spread of tuberculosis from person to person (transmission). In other words, when there is increase in the number of cases of new infection per unit of population. A mere increase in numbers of tuberculosis cases does not suggest spread. Increase in the population of the United Kingdom does not indicate an increase in the birth rate. There is compelling evidence to show that spread of tuberculosis has come to a halt in the United Kingdom. Tuberculosis in children born in this country would be proof of active tuberculosis. There is little tuberculosis in children born in the United Kingdom. Decline in tuberculosis in the population is irreversible as most of it is for reasons other than medical treatment. It began 150 years ago, a century before treatment became available.

People born more than 50 years ago had high rates of tuberculosis infection. It is that infection in the elderly that results in disease. With the passing away of the elderly population will come the end of tuberculosis in people born in the United Kingdom. Tuberculosis in native-born people reflects past experience with the infection and not its present state.

Nil rates in children accompanied by high rates in the

elderly are synonymous with imminent elimination of tuberculosis.

Prevalence of tuberculosis is confused by the very high rates of tuberculosis in people born abroad in less developed countries. Indians are the largest of this kind of community in the United Kingdom. Tuberculosis in India is now becoming stable, even declining in many areas. Infection rates, in comparison, are towards the lower end of the scale for developing countries, and there is less than one in a thousand chance for tuberculosis infection to lead to tuberculosis disease in new Indian immigrants to this country.

Reversal of the decline in tuberculosis rates in people born abroad in developing countries and now resident in the United Kingdom began twenty years ago. This coincided with massive inward movement of people from all over the developing world – previously immigrants had been mainly from the former British Asian colonies. The most important of the latest new arrival group were the black Africans.

Tuberculosis rates in Southern Africa and African Horn countries are the highest in the world. Because of the intensity of infection, the population is subject to continuous bombardment of infection and reinfection, rendering the acquired infection highly unstable. About a quarter of the children and almost the whole of the adult population eventually become infected with highly unstable infection. Their arrival in the United Kingdom is the principal cause of the increase in number of additional cases of tuberculosis in the country, reversing the previous decline. The likelihood of infection leading to disease is 10 times greater in black Africans than in Indian immigrants arriving in the country at the same time. The parts of the country where black Africans have settled, several boroughs in London and the West Midlands, are now experiencing very high rates of tuberculosis similar to those in less developed countries.

New cases of tuberculosis are not due to current transmission in the United Kingdom. Two thirds of the time the disease is imported from abroad, for the rest it is mostly the flare-up of a person's own infection contracted decades ago.

If there had been no influx of black Africans to the United Kingdom in the past ten years, there would be only a minimal imperceptible increase from the arrival of non-black Africans in the country. Only areas that have significant numbers of black Africans have shown an increase in tuberculosis; other metropolitan areas, such as Manchester and Liverpool, have continued to show either uninterrupted decline or barely noticeable increase. Most rural areas of England, Wales and Scotland are now epidemiologically free of tuberculosis. The whole of Northern Ireland is nearing elimination of tuberculosis in its entire population.

Tuberculosis is a difficult disease to contract. It needs very close social contact within individual households for the disease to have a chance to spread. Even then it fails to do so in most instances. Failure of tuberculosis to develop in children born in Britain is enough evidence of that.

A nil transmission in the childhood population, 40 cases per 100,000 in the 65+ native-born population and 1,000 to 2,000 cases per 100,000 African Horn population, notwithstanding myriad different rates in every population group, born abroad or in the United Kingdom, coupled with variable rates in successive cohorts of population, is evidence that weakens the hypothesis that 13 new cases recorded for every 100,000 population reflects the current history of tuberculosis in the country, as claimed so authoritatively by the UK government.

I provide a case study using official figures to illustrate the natural history of tuberculosis in a country in which the number of people born abroad is tiny and which typifies the epidemiology of tuberculosis in the native-born population in all developed countries, including Britain and the United States.

Northern Ireland fulfils the criteria for elimination of tuberculosis in the native-born population by the end of the first quarter of this century in 2025. It shows the progress of tuberculosis in the native-born population, uninfluenced by tuberculosis in people born abroad. The trends are similar to the whole of the United Kingdom in its native population, 94 per cent of the total.

The annual notification rate has been fewer than four cases per 100,000 population since 1990. It was 3.4 cases in the year 2003. The case rate for pulmonary (infectious) tuberculosis was only 1.6 per 100,000 population in the year 2001. Only pulmonary tuberculosis is infectious. Northern Ireland was also free of resistance to drugs, as would be largely expected in a native-born population.

In children under the age of 15 years, the case rate is now 0.6 per 100,000 population. It is near enough to a rate of one case per million children, which is an epidemiological marker for elimination of tuberculosis.

On the other end of the scale, a case rate of 13 per 100,000 elderly population reflects high exposure to infection in people when they were young. The natural decline will be accelerated exponentially as this population age group is reduced by death. Nothing can be done to hasten tuberculosis decrease in this age group. It will take its course, but will inevitably end with the demise of tuberculosis in the whole native-born population in Northern Ireland.

It is not the average case rate in a diverse population that principally predicts trends in tuberculosis, but the rate in children, as that demonstrates whether transmission is taking place. If it is not, then the cases of tuberculosis are due to reactivation of old infection in Northern Ireland. Thus a case rate of 13 per 100,000 in the elderly does not predict active tuberculosis, it is the case rate in children of 0.6 per 100,000 population which is important.

This experience is mirrored in the rest of the United Kingdom in its native-born population. The epidemiology is made complex by the tuberculosis in six per cent (six million) of the people born abroad; the elimination, however, of tuberculosis in 94 per cent (50 million) of the native-born population is irreversible.

I propose that the UK government adopt the following revised hypothesis about tuberculosis in England:

"We are pleased that transmission of tuberculosis in the United Kingdom came to a halt several years ago. The disease will be eliminated in native-born people towards the end of the first quarter of this century, when those with high rates of infection, acquired more than 50 years ago, have passed away. Meanwhile, high rates of tuberculosis are found in people born abroad in countries with high rates of the disease. In most instances, it is stable infection, and makes only a limited impact. The only exception is the very high rate of unstable tuberculosis infection in black Africans. Areas of England where black Africans have settled have experienced a dramatic rise in rates of tuberculosis, in contrast to all other areas where tuberculosis rates are either stable or decreasing.

"Even the highest rates in people born abroad have no influence on people born in this country. The spread of tuberculosis has failed to occur despite these very high exposures to tuberculosis in people born abroad in less developed countries.

"The way to maintain this fortunate state of affairs is to diagnose tuberculosis early and treat promptly all cases of the disease that arise in our elderly population from infection acquired in the distant past and in those of all ages who acquired it abroad. This policy will ensure that no spread of tuberculosis takes place in the United Kingdom. Tuberculosis is a benign disease and quickly cured – it no longer holds the terror it did in the past.

"Treatment is simple and inexpensive. Three-drugs-in-one tablets taken three times a day, at home, for six months will produce certain cure, without exception. Multiple drug resistance is less than one per cent in the country. We are adequately prepared to deal with this problem. Mostly, the patients are not ill enough to miss school or work. The treatment renders the patient non-infectious within a few days of starting treatment. There is no need to isolate a person suffering from tuberculosis once treatment is begun. There is no danger the disease will be passed to others provided treatment is administered and followed correctly.

"Immunisation and screening procedures play no part in the management of people suffering from tuberculosis. Their practice will therefore cease forthwith in this country.

"It is our intention to confirm the continuous decline in tuberculosis and zero spread of infection in England annually, as we are confident that, coupled with the natural decline, transparent and effective treatment programmes will ensure sustained control of tuberculosis until elimination is achieved in the native-born population, and sustained and durable decline in the population born abroad in less developed countries."

This hypothesis provides us with a clear statement of the natural history of tuberculosis in the United Kingdom. A plan of action based on a national focus to eliminate an eminently treatable disease follows automatically.

CHAPTER 15

Impact of Tuberculosis in London: The Making of an Epidemic

London has for centuries offered a home to immigrants. Immigrants like London and it certainly needs them. Crucial parts of the capital's infrastructure would fail without their presence.

In the United Kingdom, the number of people who arrived from less developed countries grew by 53 per cent between 1991 and 2001, and the population from 3.0 million in 1991 to 4.6 million in 2001. People from less developed countries with high prevalence of tuberculosis are concentrated in large urban centres. Nearly half (45 per cent) live in the London region where they comprise about a third of all residents. The greatest contribution to this came from black Africans, with a gain of 53 per cent in the 1991 census period and 141 per cent in the 2001 census.

Fifty per cent of all tuberculosis in the United Kingdom now occurs in London. The capital has the highest prevalence of tuberculosis in the country. By the mid-1980s fewer than 6,000 cases were reported; the number had risen to 7,000 in 2002.

The number of tuberculosis cases in any given geographical area reflects the presence of a population originating from less developed countries. London, with the highest prevalence of tuberculosis (29 per cent population from less developed countries) is followed by the West Midlands (13 per cent), the South East (eight per cent), the North West (eight per cent), Yorkshire and the Humber (eight per cent each), the North East (two per cent), and the South West (two per cent).

The prevalence of tuberculosis is uneven. The rural counties within these regions with a negligible non-native-born population have virtually no tuberculosis. Even Richmond, a London Borough, has a tuberculosis incidence of only three cases per 100,000 population. It is an example of a major urban centre with very low tuberculosis – because it has only a small non-native-born population.

Tuberculosis rates that were either stable or declining 20 years ago in the whole of the United Kingdom began to rise in those areas of the country which were receiving large numbers of immigrants.

Within this distribution of the immigrant population is the concentration of black Africans, important to the increased prevalence of tuberculosis. Areas of the country, predominantly metropolitan London and to a lesser extent Birmingham in the West Midlands, where Africans have settled are a main focus of above-average, immigrant-related tuberculosis. Most of the increase in tuberculosis in the United Kingdom in recent years is in people of African origin. Cities without an African population have not experienced a rise in tuberculosis in recent years. Africans are the most severely affected immigrant community for tuberculosis in the United Kingdom, as in the rest of Europe and the United States.

The black Africans began to arrive in significant numbers in the early 1990s. They brought in their wake unstable tuberculosis infection. The reversal of decline of tuberculosis was most dramatic and significant in London (78 per cent of the black African population) and the West Midlands (15 per cent of black Africans). The London counties and Birmingham metropolitan city, where the concentration of the black African population is the highest, have the highest rates of tuberculosis in the country. In 1987, tuberculosis cases in London accounted for fewer than 14 per cent of the national total. The figure now is 40 per cent, the highest rate of any region in England. The incidence of tuberculosis in London is now three times higher than the national average rate. The United Kingdom tuberculosis rate increased from 8.4 per 100,000 population in 1988 to 9.2 per 100,000 population in 1993. This increase paralleled the increase of the black African population in London and Birmingham.

Seventy-five per cent of tuberculosis notifications are in people born abroad, of which the black Africans show the greatest increase. Seventy-seven cases recorded in black Africans in 1988 increased to 1,401 in 2002. Tuberculosis rates in areas with the highest African population are 40.9 per 100,000 population for London and 15.6 per 100,000 population for the West Midlands. The rate for the country is 12.9 per 100,000 population. If it were not for the input of tuberculosis from black Africans, tuberculosis rates would have shown a continuous fall in all areas of the country, including London and Birmingham, as was happening two decades earlier.

Of the 33 London boroughs, 12, with a substantial non-native-born population, have above average tuberculosis rates. The highest rates of tuberculosis in London are recorded in the boroughs of Newham, Tower Hamlets and Brent, which have the highest concentration of black Africans living in London.

This is in contrast to the rate of tuberculosis in the Indian population, the largest ethnic minority group in London. The rates slowed down from 38 per 100,000 population between 1981 and 1991 to 27 per 100,000 population between 1991 and 2001, as a result of stable rates of tuberculosis in India from where most of the Indians came. Over a similar period, London boroughs with a high concentration of Indians, but with low density of black Africans, have shown only a slight increase in tuberculosis, despite the arrival of immigrant Indians sometimes in greater numbers than black Africans. Examples are the London boroughs of Ealing, Hounslow and Wembley.

A similar impact on rates of tuberculosis with the arrival of black Africans has been noticed in several other European countries and the United States.

Not all London areas are affected. Those without residents born in African countries (Havering, Bromley, Kingston, and Richmond) have continued their uninterrupted decline in tuberculosis, as has rest of the country, except Birmingham and a few other metropolitan areas which have also seen increase in numbers because of the increase in number of new residents born abroad, especially in Africa.

The rates of tuberculosis in the African Horn population are quoted as varying from 1,200 to 2,000 per 100,000 population in studies conducted in Europe and the United States. In the West Midlands region of England, the number of cases in black Africans doubled in one year, from 2002 to 2003, with rates quoted as 760 per 100,000 population. This compares to the next highest rate of 100 cases per 100,000 population in people of South Asian origin and the lowest in the Afro-Caribbean community at 15 cases per 100,000 population (see Table 5).

Table 5 Estimates of tuberculosis burden in the highest incidence countries with migration links to the UK (This information was obtained from WHO sources. Experience in the United Kingdom and elsewhere in Europe and the United States shows that the rates for African countries though high are still underestimated).

Country	Population (000s)	Incidence cases (000s)	Rate per 100,000
Asia			
India	960,178	1,799	187
China	1,243,738	1,402	113
Pakistan	143,831	261	181
Africa			
Nigeria	118,369	253	214
South Africa	336	170	
Ethiopia	60,148	156	260
DRC	48,040	129	269
Tanzania	31,507	97	308
Kenya	28,414	84	297
Uganda	20,791	66	320
Zimbabwe	11,682	63	538

In Seattle, USA, the annual number of tuberculosis cases among Africans increased threefold from 1993–1997 to 1998–2001. Of 71 cases in Africans, 32 (45 per cent) occurred within one year after arrival, and 60 (65 per cent) occurred within five years. This indicates that Africans were carrying unstable infection when arriving in the host country and attests to the intensity of infection in the country of origin. Similarly, in the West Midlands metropolitan counties, a quarter of all cases were in people who had arrived in the country less than five years ago.

Most black African immigrants are young. Tuberculosis prevalence is highest among young adults between 15 and 24 years of age. Black African children contributed most to childhood tuberculosis in London. In 1998, 44 per cent (23 per cent in 1993) of children with tuberculosis were black Africans. The most common country of origin was Somalia, with the highest rates of tuberculosis in the world. Sixty-six per cent of the African children were born abroad and developed tuberculosis within five years of arrival in London, no doubt reactivation of unstable infection acquired abroad.

Added to all this is the high birth rate in immigrants including black Africans. There were 104,200 live births (with 58,600 deaths) in London in 2001, a natural population growth of 45,600. Natural population growth in London accounted for 70 per cent of the total natural growth of the United Kingdom population in 2001, even though London was home to only 29 per cent of the total immigrant population.

The rate of tuberculosis in most sub-Saharan African countries exceeds 600 cases per 100,000 population. Estimates of 1,200 to 2,000 cases per 100,000 population have been made in the Somali population settled in European countries and the United States. Such prevalence of tuberculosis will give rise to continuous infection and reinfection in the population starting from birth. One in two persons including children (50 per cent) will be expected to bring in this infection when they arrive in the United Kingdom. The prevalence of infection will approach 100 per cent in Somali born adults, the people with the highest rates of tuberculosis in the world. The infection they carry is mostly unstable, and will result in disease much more often than in other populations. Tuberculosis will occur in one in 10 Somali-born people, especially children, within five years of arrival in the United Kingdom, compared with one in a hundred in Indian born children. The statement that tuberculosis occurs within five years of arrival in the United Kingdom speaks for the instability of the infection in the African-born population. Further, that it occurs in children is evidence of the tuberculosis epidemic in Somalia where the entire adult population appears to be infected.

Such an intense load of unstable infection in black Africans is the cause of dramatic reversal of decline in tuberculosis in London and Birmingham where black Africans are predominantly settled.

In a review of tuberculosis epidemiology by the London Assembly Health Committee, it was stated that tuberculosis was a complex disease:

"Treatment of the disease was complicated by social factors. Social deprivation and marginalisation had a major impact on the transmission; those who were socially marginalized were those who were most vulnerable to the disease. Tuberculosis is, and always has been, a disease engendered by poverty. Social and economic deprivation, particularly bad housing, is a breeding ground for *Mycobacterium tuberculosis.*"

This is a mumbo-jumbo theory of an infectious disease and its causes. Some of the poorest and most deprived rural areas in the United Kingdom have no tuberculosis because they are not exposed to it and have no non-white people settled among them. Afro-Caribbeans, perhaps even more deprived than black Africans economically, do not suffer from tuberculosis. It is not without irony that the London Assembly Health Committee goes on to praise New York for having brought a quick halt to its epidemic after having spent over a billion dollars to do so.

Seattle, one of the richest cities in the United States, was free of tuberculosis until there was a huge influx of black African immigrants, especially Somali-born people. The city now competes with, and may even exceed, London in its prevalence of tuberculosis.

The principle of tuberculosis control is to prevent the spread from one person to another. Spread is halted by early diagnosis and treatment of the disease. The problem with control of tuberculosis lies not in its medical treatment but in its entanglement with spurious social and economic factors, as in London, losing sight of the fact that it is an infectious disease, curable with cheap and readily available drugs.

No assault on poverty or deprivation will ever bring tuberculosis under control. Immigrants may no longer be poor but they will still suffer from tuberculosis if the disease is not treated.

PART FIVE

Vaccination

CHAPTER 16

BCG Vaccination

Over 100 million children worldwide receive BCG vaccination every year. But the protective effect of BCG vaccination is uncertain because of the wide variations in effectiveness found in different trials worldwide. Despite universal usage for over 50 years, it is still not possible to demonstrate its influence on tuberculosis morbidity. No unequivocal beneficial effects have been demonstrated for vaccination after the age of one year. The three studies of BCG vaccination for children older than one year of age show a poor level of protection, less than 30 per cent. The protective effect of BCG vaccination is one of hope rather than fact. BCG differs from other vaccines whose impact is well-established and unchallenged.

Neither the relevance of BCG vaccination to a person who is vaccinated nor its influence on the population in which the vaccination takes place is defined. Protective efficacy is a measure of the proportion of people who would have contracted the disease had they not had the vaccination. Such efficacy is not demonstrated for BCG vaccine. Its protective effect, if any, in developed countries is now so small that it can no longer be quantified. Its status is more of a political device to assuage public fear than of medical benefit.

In the United Kingdom, the national policy is to offer BCG

vaccination to adolescents who are at additional risk of developing tuberculosis. Of the very few studies in school children, the largest ever carried out was in India. Not only was there no protection, the study actually appeared to suggest harm from vaccination.

A trial carried out in the 1950s in the United Kingdom is the only evidence we have of protection approaching 80 per cent in this age group. Yet this trial was carried out with a non-BCG vaccine. The results of the trial have never been reproduced elsewhere. Following its only trial in the UK, the use of the vaccine was abandoned. It is a measure of desperation to show the benefits of vaccinating children that we rely on this 50-year old trial with a non-BCG vaccine to justify vaccination of children. There is now universal agreement that vaccinating adolescent or older people is not a useful intervention.

The WHO recommends that BCG vaccination be offered only to newborn infants to avoid serious forms of the disease in countries with high rates of tuberculosis. The International Union Against Tuberculosis and Lung Disease (IUATLD) concludes that BCG vaccination cannot be expected to have any impact on the epidemiological situation of tuberculosis even in countries with very high rates of the disease.

The US, Holland and Sweden, countries with the lowest prevalence of tuberculosis in the world, do not use BCG vaccination. There is no discernible effect on childhood and teenage tuberculosis. The disease is absent in these age groups.

BCG (Bacillus Calmette Guérin) vaccine contains live but weakened *Mycobacterium bovis*, bacteria that are closely related to human *Mycobacterium tuberculosis*. *Mycobacterium bovis* causes natural infection in cattle and in human beings who drink unpasteurised, infected milk. Different BCG vaccines are available worldwide, but they are all derived from the original *Mycobacterium bovis* strain.

BCG vaccine produces localised infection at the site of the vaccination. The vaccine also induces hypersensitivity similar to that produced by natural infection. The vaccine is expected to confer protection against tuberculosis, as is supposed does the natural infection.

BCG-vaccinated persons develop positive reactions to tuberculin skin test, a reaction similar to that produced by the natural infection. However, the relationship between vaccine-induced protection and sensitivity is not consistent, giving rise to uncertainty about the nature of its protectiveness, as tuberculin skin test reactivity (hypersensitivity) does not correspond to the degree of effectiveness or its protection from tuberculosis. The size does not indicate strength of protection.

Tuberculin reactivity caused by BCG vaccination produces a tuberculin skin test reaction indistinguishable from that of natural infection. In practice, the BCG-induced tuberculin skin test reaction ranges from no indurations to a moderate reaction at the skin test site. The size of a tuberculin skin reaction in a BCG-vaccinated person is not a factor in determining whether there is natural tuberculosis infection or an effect due to the vaccination itself.

The relation between the duration and size of a post-BCG vaccination tuberculin skin test reaction and the duration and strength of protection against tuberculosis remains undefined. Modern molecular technology suggests that the test reaction, whatever the size, has no proportional link to protectiveness.

The precise duration of BCG vaccination-induced immunity is not certain. Too little is known about it. The period of protection is claimed to range from five to 15 years. The British study quoted above found that protectiveness falls rapidly after 10 years. Lack of accurate information on duration of BCG vaccine efficacy has important implications regarding the reliability of estimates of the impact of BCG vaccination on the outcome of the disease.

Our current understanding is that the presence or absence of a positive tuberculin test response after BCG vaccination does not directly or proportionally reflect protective efficacy. The size of a post-vaccination tuberculin skin test reaction does not predict whether or not BCG will provide protection against tuberculosis.

The aim of BCG vaccination is to mimic tuberculosis infection and prevent further re-infection, reducing the opportunity for infection to progress to disease by inducing immunity. It does not itself prevent infection from taking place. Prevention of tuberculosis disease breaks the chain of transmission to stop spread. Only 10 per cent of natural infection ever progresses to disease. The impact of BCG vaccination will be on this 10 per cent and not the whole infected population. The number of infected people in low prevalence countries is small; the annual risk of infection is less than 0.01 per cent. The influence of BCG vaccination will be minimal, even to the extent that it may not be recordable.

The fact that the accepted BCG protective efficacy is 10 years means that protection disappears in children vaccinated at birth when they enter their adolescence. It will be young adulthood for those similarly vaccinated in the school programme in the teenage years. Every study ever carried out on the benefits of BCG vaccination is unanimous in accepting that it has no effect in preventing pulmonary disease.

In infants, the annual risk of infection is less than 0.01 per cent. One per cent of infected infants develop tuberculosis meningitis. If 100,000 infants are vaccinated with BCG with an average 50 per cent protective effect, then 100 children become infected of whom one will develop meningitis. This is prevention of one case of tuberculosis meningitis in the United Kingdom when 100,000 children are vaccinated. Other estimates suggest one case of meningitis prevented per one million children vaccinated. The latter estimate is made in the light of a very dramatic drop of infection in children under the age of five in recent years in the United States.

However, DNA molecular technology has thrown doubts on the premise that infection protects against re-infection, the assumption on which the protectiveness of BCG vaccination is based. The DNA molecular studies show that re-infection occurs in proportion to the intensity of infection in the population. The failure of natural infection to protect against re-infection explains the ineffectiveness of BCG vaccination. BCG vaccination must influence cellular immunity in order to provide protection. Cellular immunity depends on tubercular sensitivity. If tubercular sensitivity is not a factor in protection from the disease, then the basis of BCG vaccination is undermined.

Tuberculin test class 1 reactions are assumed to be negative and class 2 reactions protective in those with a previous history of vaccination. A class 2 reaction in the absence of vaccination is positive for infection. These, however, are arbitrary interpretations and not based on fact.

In the absence of known correlates of protective immunity, the assumption that BCG-induced tuberculin sensitivity provides a measure of protection must be recognised as untrue. Strong tuberculin-sensitivity is associated with high risk of disease. Progressive tuberculin sensitivity represents aggressive immunological activity in the host. The stronger the reaction, the less likely it is to be to the benefit of the host. Most authorities insist that the presence of tuberculin sensitivity is essential to protectiveness and claim that a low degree of tuberculin sensitivity is more protective than a higher degree. The authorities provide no evidence for this assertion. In people who have no history of contact with a case of tuberculosis in a low prevalence country, such sensitivity is more likely to be evidence of cross-reacting, non-tuberculosis antigens than tuberculosis itself (false positive). Even more important is the fact that a weak reaction is no guarantee that infection will not proceed to active disease.

Tuberculosis in children is not infectious. Vaccination in

children has no effect on the rate of infection and does not reduce transmission of the disease. BCG vaccination does not prevent infection.

BCG is the most popular vaccine in the less developed world, yet tuberculosis remains the commonest serious disease in children. Despite lack of evidence of its effectiveness enthusiasm for its use remains undiminished.

Vaccination in adolescence does not reduce the risk of developing pulmonary tuberculosis. The World Health Organisation recommends the use of BCG vaccine only in infancy to prevent serious childhood forms of tuberculosis (meningitis, progressive and miliary tuberculosis). The main burden of the disease is pulmonary disease in adults. BCG has no influence on the infectious form of tuberculosis and hence its transmission. If the clinical efficacy is measured in terms of the percentage reduction in disease among vaccinated individuals, then the claimed protective efficacy rates, which range from two per cent to 80 per cent for prevention of tuberculosis and 52 per cent to 100 per cent for prevention of tuberculosis meningitis and miliary tuberculosis, increase uncertainty about the value of the vaccination.

Several major and influential studies have produced negative effects. More tuberculosis is seen among those receiving the vaccine than in the controls not receiving the vaccine. No random, controlled population studies have ever been carried out to assess the effectiveness of BCG vaccination in children.

In developed countries, the serious forms of tuberculosis in children have become so rare that 100,000 to 1,000,000 infants would need to be vaccinated to prevent one case of the serious form of the disease. An infant who is a close contact of a case of tuberculosis is treated for tuberculosis to eliminate risk of infection, regardless of vaccination status. This makes BCG vaccination during infancy unnecessary.

The protective efficacy of BCG vaccination has been marred by its uncertainty since its launch in the mid-20th century. There is a great variation in results of clinical trials of BCG vaccination in different parts of the world. Various explanations are offered for the extraordinary variability of BCG protection. Two plausible explanations are the powerful secular downward trend, and the dramatic decline in the disease with treatment overwhelming the effect of the vaccine, but erroneously attributed to it.

We lack current evidence of the level of efficacy of BCG vaccination of children. The most recent trials of efficacy are decades old. The natural history of tuberculosis has changed remarkably since then and no longer corresponds to the parameters of old studies. Most of these studies have been found to have design faults and would no longer be acceptable today.

The principal recommendations for BCG vaccination in the United Kingdom were set out more than 50 years ago. A dual vaccination policy is practised. Infants born to mothers at "high risk", invariably non-white, are given BCG at birth. Children in their early teen years, usually of non-white origin, are offered BCG vaccination if not vaccinated at birth. Risk of tuberculosis is principally related to country of birth not race. Children whose parents were born in this country have no greater risk of infection irrespective of their racial origin.

The rationale for the programme in the teen years is to make use of the 10-year duration of vaccination immunity in order to prevent disease among young adults, in whom pulmonary tuberculosis was common when BCG vaccination was first introduced 50 years ago. This is no longer so and tuberculosis is rare at this age. We also know now that BCG vaccination does not prevent pulmonary tuberculosis.

BCG is not given to children who bear a previous BCG scar. This is most often in children of non-white origin, vaccinated at birth. As tuberculosis is expected to be more common in such children as they grow up into young adulthood, this policy defies its own purpose. The very children who need BCG vaccination in adolescence, whose neonatal BCG protective immunity has waned by this time, are the ones who are denied it.

The implications of a post-vaccination scar for protection against disease are undetermined, as there is no evidence of a relationship between scar size or its absence following vaccination and protection against tuberculosis. The policy that vaccination is only offered once in a lifetime creates a conflict in its availability at birth or early teenage years. The fact that tuberculosis is not found at either age makes the conflict irrelevant. The use of the vaccination itself at any age is unjustified.

The reason for vaccinating infants born to mothers at "high

risk" (in other words non-white women) of tuberculosis is also not valid, as these babies have not been shown to be at a higher risk of tuberculosis or of developing the more serious forms of the disease. It is not known why non-white mothers born and resident in this country are considered at high risk of tuberculosis. The spread of tuberculosis is the same in all mothers, as is the case for children born irrespective of the antecedents of their parents or their vaccination status when comparison is made with countries which do not offer BCG vaccination.

In 1950, it was necessary to vaccinate 67 school children with BCG to prevent one case of tuberculosis; it was 3,600 vaccinations in 1989 and 15,000 in 1999. The figure will have risen to between 50,000 to 100,000 vaccinated children in the year 2005 to prevent one case of tuberculosis.

It is difficult to quantify potential benefits of BCG vaccination. BCG has failed to reduce tuberculosis in adults. The problem in tuberculosis is delayed or failed diagnosis coupled with failed or inadequate treatment owing to lack of anti-tuberculosis drugs or inappropriate management of the disease. No amount of BCG vaccination will compensate for this deficiency.

We will now consider the confusion in differentiating between reactivity to the tuberculin skin test following vaccination and natural infection. BCG vaccination hinders investigation of transmission after exposure to tuberculosis and the effective treatment of infection.

It is not possible to tell the difference between a positive test due to BCG vaccination and one due to natural infection with tuberculosis.

Countries which use BCG vaccination believe it is possible to do so on the basis of the degree of the size of the reaction following a tuberculin skin test. Since the explanation for the degree of the reaction size is in doubt such claims are questionable. The United States does not use BCG partly for the reason that it is not possible to make such a distinction.

Without BCG, tuberculin test induced sensitivity facilitates the use of the test for contact investigation, source identification and selection of individuals for treatment of infection. By confounding the tuberculin skin test, BCG vaccination nullifies the only practical tool to establish infection and initiate treatment. In the United Kingdom, confusion in the interpretation of a test reaction where there is a previous history of BCG vaccination militates against the effective management necessary to prevent transmission of tuberculosis.

BCG vaccination exposes children to an unnecessary medical procedure. What is more, BCG vaccination can have significant adverse effects.

BCG is the most reactogenic childhood vaccine in use. It is the only commonly used vaccine to induce a local skin inflammatory response that persists for several weeks, even months.

The local lesion begins as a papule, two or more weeks after vaccination. It then proceeds to a painful ulceration. The ulcer heals after several weeks leaving an ugly, prominent depressed pigmented scar on the site of the vaccination. The local lymph nodes often develop accompanying palpable painful swellings. These reactions are considered the "normal" response to the vaccination. The unsightly blemish is a useful, if imperfect, indication of past BCG vaccination.

Abscesses at the site of BCG vaccination are common. Deep, sloughing abscesses result in painful inflammation of draining lymph nodes. The inflamed nodes may break down to open wounds on to the skin surface. These take a long time to heal. Rarely, spread of BCG infection results in systemic complications including inflammation in the spleen, liver, kidney and bladder and bones.

Generalised common adverse effects of the vaccine are headaches, fever and enlargement of regional lymph nodes.

In addition, there is a wide range of adverse conditions related to the hypersensitive effect of the vaccination because of reactions to the live bacteria in the vaccine. These include rashes, widespread skin reactions and inflammation of the eyes. Allergic reactions, including anaphylactic shock, may also occur. Disseminated infection and shock due to hypersensitive reaction are the most serious. Studies in Sweden show a one in 1,000 to a one in 10,000 chance for disseminated BCG complications, such as infection of the bones, to occur in some vaccinated populations. This was the major reason that BCG vaccination was stopped in Sweden as serious harmful effects outweighed the benefits.

BCG is difficult to administer as an intradermal injection at any age, but especially so to a newborn. The commonest mistake is to give the injection too deep, failing to raise the classical orange-skin appearance in the dermis. Local injection site abscesses may occur, typically as a result of improper injection technique when the vaccine is given into the subcutaneous layers of the skin. Outbreaks of BCG vaccination reactions are not uncommon, manifested as large ulcers and local lymphadenopathy. Keloid formation at the scar site appears to be more common in some, for example, African and Asian, populations than in others. Most of the adverse effects of tuberculosis are not notified as these are regarded as normal reactions to the vaccine.

PART SIX

Screening

CHAPTER 17

Ionising Radiation in Screening for Tuberculosis

The Ionising Radiation (Medical Exposure) Regulations 2000 (Health and Safety 2000 N0 1059) apply to the following medical exposures:

A. The exposure of patients as part of their own medical diagnosis or treatment.
B. The exposure of individuals as part of health screening programmes.

The regulations stipulate that no person shall carry out a medical exposure unless it has been justified as showing a sufficient net benefit and that in the case of a female of childbearing age, pregnancy or breastfeeding have been taken into account.

The regulations require that the specific objectives of the exposure and the characteristics of the individual involved have been considered, including the total potential diagnostic or therapeutic benefits, and that the direct health benefit to the individual and the benefit to society of the exposure are assured. They require that the efficacy, benefit and risk of available alternative techniques having the same objective but involving no exposure to ionising radiation have been taken into account.

In considering the weight to be given to the above matters in justifying an exposure, the practitioner must pay special attention to (a) medical exposures as part of a health screening programme, (b) medical exposure of children (under 18 years of age), and (c) the urgency of the exposure in cases involving (i) a female in whom pregnancy cannot be excluded and (ii) a female who is breastfeeding.

Clinical evaluation of the outcome of each medical exposure is recorded, including procedures for making enquiries of females of childbearing age to establish whether they are or may be pregnant or breastfeeding.

Under these regulations, a practitioner takes responsibility for individual medical exposure of patients as part of their own medical diagnosis or treatment, and the exposure of individuals as part of health screening.

The regulations prohibit practitioners from carrying out a medical exposure in the case of a female of childbearing age in whom it has been established without doubt that she is pregnant or breastfeeding.

There is a wide variation in absorbed doses in patients. Radiography of the chest is the most commonly performed procedure in adults. The risk of radiation exposure to the patient is usually small for any one procedure, but pregnant women need special consideration. In the screening setting, it is not really possible to obtain adequate information, especially history of a missed period and recent radiological exposure. Radiological procedures should not be performed as an alternative to taking a thorough history and physical examination.

The referral of a patient for chest X-ray should provide an accurate and rapid diagnosis, which enables the most efficacious steps to be taken to benefit the person in terms of treatment. Over-utilisation of radiology results in an unnecessary radiation burden to the community. If a request is inappropriate, the radiologist should refuse to undertake the radiographic procedure.

In the absence of clear clinical indications, it is unlikely that radiological procedures will demonstrate the pathological condition requiring treatment. Ionising radiation in such circumstances is not justified. Examination using ionising radiation should be undertaken only if the findings are likely to affect the management of the patient. Another problem with screening of asymptomatic patients is that inconclusive results lead to a cycle of repeat X-rays, taken to confirm findings in those submitted from the screening centre.

Nevertheless in the case of tuberculosis and immigration there is a demand for more procedures, not a reduction.

CHAPTER 18

Screening of Immigrants

Increased immigration from less developed countries has led to calls for pre-entry tuberculosis screening to be introduced for immigrants to the United Kingdom. These proposals seem to be grounded in common sense. If there is an increase in immigration and a related increase in tuberculosis, the government needs to introduce measures to protect the public from imported disease. Its failure to do so will be seen as "standing silently on the politically correct sidelines".

Screening is the systematic application of a medical test to a defined population. Screening appeals to policy makers because of their wish to be seen to be "doing something" about a health problem. It appears to be a sensible step to take. Screening, though, is not always a universal panacea to limit an infectious disease. It is certainly not in the case of tuberculosis.

Disease screening is one of the most basic tools of preventive medicine. Screening programmes have a long history in efforts to control epidemics of infectious diseases. Screening has an intuitive appeal. It brings forward the diagnosis. Earlier diagnosis benefits the patient by early treatment and the public by preventing spread. Screening of intending immigrants in the country of origin or destination is considered a valid tool for limiting the spread of tuberculosis in host countries.

The purpose of screening is two-fold: to identify individuals who will benefit from prompt treatment; and to protect the host community by identifying individuals with infectious tuberculosis and stop them from spreading the disease.

Two methods allow for screening of tuberculosis:

Tuberculin skin test
The skin test detects infection. Only 10 per cent of infection ever proceeds to disease. Treating everyone with detected infection will be a mammoth task, and unrewarding, as nine tenths of the infection-positive people treated would never develop the disease anyway. The tuberculin skin test is not used for routine screening of asymptomatic people.

Chest X-ray screening
This is the universal method adopted for screening immigrants from less developed countries. Under United Kingdom legislation, immigration officers have the right to refer persons who are seeking to enter and settle in the country to government approved medical inspectors for screening for tuberculosis.

Under the obligatory UK immigration policy, immigrants seeking domicile for settlement, work or study from any country with an annual incidence of tuberculosis of more than 40 cases per 100,000 population – that is, all the less developed countries – are required to undergo chest X-ray examination.

Of the entry ports to the United Kingdom, only London

Heathrow Airport Health Control Unit has chest X-ray facilities on site; indeed it is the only port of entry in the world to do so. Immigrants requiring chest X-rays from all other ports of entry are referred to the medical facilities in the area of intended residence. Children, who bear the heaviest burden of tuberculosis in less developed countries, are exempt from chest X-ray examinations.

Screening for disease (active case finding) by mass radiography was a common practice in the past. However, chest X-ray screening for tuberculosis has been abandoned because of low yield and high cost. Chest X-rays are inefficient in screening for tuberculosis in persons without symptoms. The detection rate is less than 0.05 per cent in persons screened. X-Ray equipment is expensive to buy and maintain and it requires specially trained doctors and technicians to operate the machines and interpret the results – the whole package amounting to a high material expense. It costs over £100,000 to detect one case of infectious tuberculosis in asymptomatic new arrivals at the London Heathrow Health Control Unit. A reason why screening for tuberculosis is inappropriate is that the actual number of cases at any one time is low, despite it being one of the most serious infectious diseases in the world, and sometimes the commonest cause of death in young and middle-aged persons.

There is no evidence that screening of immigrants has an influence on the incidence of tuberculosis in the host country. The effect of screening on reducing person-time of infectiousness, and the number of cases of disease averted by early detection are not quantified by any country enforcing this method, even after decades of screening of immigrants. It is not known how much tuberculosis is uncovered in immigrants screened in the country of their origin.

Despite lack of evidence for effectiveness, many countries continue to practise chest X-ray screening for immigrants. Taking the tuberculosis case rate as 40 per 100,000 population, 900,960 of 100,000 people undergoing radiography will be free of the disease. Of the 40 cases detected, less than a third would be infectious.

The high prevalence of tuberculosis among new arrivals seems to imply a risk of transmission of infection to the host population. This has proved not to be the case. The main reason for screening on entry – to prevent spread of tuberculosis – is not valid in the light of the evidence.

Compliance with screening is poor in all developed countries even when backed with rigorous legal or administrative requirements. The problem is that few sanctions can be applied to a person who does not comply with the screening policy in a free and democratic country. Ensuring compliance with screening in a free country is a daunting task. The lack of success results in little effort being devoted to follow-up of recalcitrant immigrants. Most countries requiring screening report a compliance rate of less than 50 per cent for entry screening once the new arrivals are in the country. Compliance is much lower for any person needing follow-up visits.

Experience from other countries requiring entry screening for immigrants has been discouraging. Studies in Australia report unsatisfactorily high proportions of immigrants (27 per cent and 60 per cent respectively) from high prevalence countries who fail to comply with screening.

Evaluations of effectiveness of screening and data on follow-up and outcome must be collected and analysed systematically. The information is necessary for rational decision-making on optimal frequency and duration of screening. No such information is available – it is difficult to envisage that a nationwide information system on the coverage and yield of screening would be available, and indeed none is.

No developed country, by the very nature of its governance, has a complete registration system for entry or exit follow-up of its people, be they citizens, legitimate immigrants, refugees, asylum seekers, illegal entrants, seasonal workers or students. A system for identifying new immigrants at high risk for tuberculosis needs to be in place, but how this is to be achieved except by making oppressive laws for the whole country is difficult to see.

If such information is not available, can we rely on our intuition to believe that benefit accrues? Epidemiology of tuberculosis allows for no such inference. Influence of screening on the prevalence of tuberculosis in the native-born or immigrant sections of the population in developed countries cannot be anticipated.

In a study of 96,638 new arrivals at London Heathrow airport, 51 persons with positive cultures were identified. The annual notification rate of persons with positive cultures in 1979 in the resident Indian and Pakistani populations was 136 per 100,000. Far fewer cases were being detected at Heathrow Airport Health Control Unit than were notified in the comparable ethnic groups resident in Britain. Yet routine screening of residents is not carried out. In British Columbia, Canada, of 21,959 newly arrived immigrants between 1982 and 1985, the number of tuberculosis cases that had been discovered by the end of the study was more in those with normal chest X-rays than in those with abnormal ones. A comprehensive review of all studies on screening supports these findings.

Chest X-ray screening is wasteful of resources and results in unnecessary radiation from millions of chest X-rays carried out over the years in developed countries. No radiographic examination should ever be permitted, for ethical and legal reasons, unless it is of proven benefit to the person undergoing examination. The fact that the number of cases of disease uncovered is lower than those notified in the settled immigrant population raises the question, "Why, if screening is of benefit, is the whole immigrant population not subjected to it?"

For screening of tuberculosis to be effective it must detect those with the condition in such a way that it assists in achieving the desired control. Systematic screening for tuberculosis on a large scale has been practised in the countries of origin (pre-screening) and arrival (post-screening) by the United States, Australia and New Zealand for over 50 years. Such screening has conspicuously failed to make an impact on the number of tuberculosis cases related to migration in those countries.

None of the immigrant screening programmes in any of the developed countries has ever been assessed against criteria of effectiveness of screening. No randomised controlled trials have been performed. Indeed the screening programmes amount to its occasional case detection rather than a cohesive outcome to control tuberculosis.

If screening does not contribute to control of tuberculosis, does then occasional detection make setting up a screening programme worthwhile when a single case actively detected would cost hundreds of times more than a case detected passively as the disease arises in the community?

The continuing practice of screening reflects ignorance of epidemiology of the disease, or deliberate disregard of the outcome of the process because of political demands. Screening of immigrants is ineffective but it will not stop governments introducing programmes of screening if they see political advantage is to be gained, irrespective of the cost or outcome.

Before a screening programme is introduced universally, evidence of the risks posed, effectiveness of intervention and economic costs are considered. Screening programmes are always expensive; the costs must be set against benefits. These have never been demonstrated for tuberculosis.

Tuberculosis does not of course discriminate between asylum seekers and other immigrants who wish to settle in the country. Indeed, asylum seekers are no more responsible for increase in tuberculosis than any other category of immigrants. Tuberculosis rates are linked to the rates of tuberculosis in the country of origin; they are relatively high if the origin is a less developed country and equal or even lower if the origin is another developed country. Politically defined asylum seekers and legal settlers (for example spouses and children) may come from countries with high or low rates of tuberculosis. Distinction between an asylum seeker and another category of immigrant wishing to settle is not epidemiologically valid.

Calculations show that the yield of infectious tuberculosis will always be low on chest X-ray screening. Of the 41,470 asylum seekers who had chest X-rays between 1995 and 1999 at London Heathrow Airport Health Control Centre 100 were found to have pulmonary tuberculosis, of which only 24 had the infectious form. In this study, the prevalence of pulmonary tuberculosis in asylum seekers was 241 per 100,000 population. However, these rates were substantially lower than rates in the same communities in London. The actual number of cases detected during screening only represented a small proportion of annually notified cases (less than 0.5 per cent) in the country.

The issue of screening new arrivals in the United Kingdom has been principally focused, for political reasons, on asylum seekers. Most asylum seekers do not use Heathrow airport to enter the country. Only Heathrow airport possesses X-ray facilities. In the year 2002, 55,276 asylum seekers arrived in the United Kingdom through Heathrow airport as compared with 169,029 legal immigrants. The incompleteness of the system does not reflect well on the national screening programme for asylum seekers.

The focusing of screening programmes on only a small proportion of immigrants to the United Kingdom, such as asylum seekers, means that other immigrants at greater or equal risk of disease are not screened. The limited impact of such measures is exacerbated if screening programmes are only available at a single point of entry and if arrival at other ports of entry means that most of these individuals do not undergo screening. For example, one study estimated that less than one quarter of immigrants to the United Kingdom are traced and screened for tuberculosis. Another study showed that port of arrival systems failed to identify 60 per cent of new immigrants to one area of the United Kingdom.

Most immigrants who are going to develop the disease do so after they have entered the country, often decades later. A study in the Netherlands, which investigated the occurrence of pulmonary disease in asylum seekers, found the rate to be high on entry, at 222 per 100,000 population. The incidence of pulmonary tuberculosis within one year after entry was estimated at 173 per 100,000. That is, the numbers of cases detected on entry were almost equivalent to those detected a year later.

The purpose of screening is to prevent spread. If there were no screening, to what degree would immigrant-associated tuberculosis pose a threat to the public? How much disease would result as a consequence of transmission from recently arrived immigrant populations?

Transmission of tuberculosis in the native-born population is rare. For instance, in the United States, a study showed very little correlation between tuberculosis rates in foreign-born and US-born populations. The states with high levels of tuberculosis in foreign-born individuals did not have high rates in those born in the United States. Immigrant-associated tuberculosis was not contributing to the burden of disease in the population born in the host country. The assertion that a considerable amount of time must pass before the impact of higher prevalence of the disease in immigrant populations is seen is disproved by the fact that immigrants have been in the country for over 50 years without cross-transmission ever having taken place. Instead rates in the US-born population have continued to decline without interruption, independently of rates in the foreign-born population.

DNA fingerprint studies in London assessed the degree of recent transmission that occurred in the city. The study found that even in immigrants only 14 per cent of cases of tuberculosis resulted from recent transmission, the rest were caused by reactivation from infection acquired years earlier in the country of origin. There was no transmission to native-born people. Other recent studies show that even transmission among immigrants is rare, leaving only reactivation of disease to be considered in the design of appropriate treatment programmes for introduction in the immigrant community.

A Danish study revealed that transmission between immigrants and individuals born in Denmark was nearly non-existent. This is the experience in those regions of the United Kingdom where treatment facilities are available to all residents including immigrants.

Synopsis of studies on screening

1. The London Heathrow Airport Health Control Unit

carried out 149,000 routine inspections under the immigration laws in 2002 and 2003; of these, 57,000 received a chest X-ray. The number of cases of pulmonary tuberculosis was 91; of these 18 were infectious cases (19 per cent). The incidence of infectious tuberculosis was 0.03 per cent or 31 per 100,000 population. Over 50 health care staff, numerous immigration and airport security and general officers were engaged in an elaborate exercise to unearth 18 new arrivals suffering from infectious tuberculosis.

2. In an analysis of 20,000 chest X-rays carried out at London Heathrow airport, an infectious disease rate of 0.1 per cent was recorded.

3. In a review of 407 chest X-ray examinations of new arrivals in Birmingham, United Kingdom, during 2000 and 2001, no active case of tuberculosis was diagnosed. An audit of 226 cases in 1992 had also showed no active tuberculosis. No case of sputum positive tuberculosis has been identified in the newly arrived in the past 10 years in the city. Birmingham is the largest recipient of immigrants outside London. Of the 126 persons with chest X-ray abnormalities, referred for further screening by the London Heathrow Airport Health Control Unit during 1983 to 1985, only two culture positive cases and no direct sputum smear positive cases were recorded.

4. A study of 1,691 and 2,242 new arrivals between 1983–1988 and 1990–1994 showed 0.65 per cent and 0.45 per cent respectively with active tuberculosis in Blackburn, United Kingdom.

5. In Croydon, United Kingdom, screening of 2,855 new

entrants resulted in the detection of three cases of tuberculosis. One hundred and ten cases of active tuberculosis were notified by passive case finding in the community during the same period.

CHAPTER 19

Effectiveness of Chest X-Rays as a Screening Tool for Tuberculosis

Chest X-rays are the principal tools used to screen for tuberculosis at ports of entry. They are the most ineffective way of screening for active disease in persons without symptoms. The question of accuracy of the tool used to detect active disease is critical to the value of a screening test. Screening tests indicate a high or low probability of disease, not its definitive presence, and misclassifications are inevitable. In order to understand whether chest X-rays might be useful as screening tools we need to understand the three principles of sensitivity, specificity and positive predictive value.

Sensitivity is the probability that the disease will be shown to be present with the test. Specificity is the probability that an individual will test negative if the disease is absent. Positive predictive value is the probability that an individual actually has the disease if the test is positive; it is dependent on the sensitivity and specificity of the screening test, and also the prevalence – the proportion of the population that has disease. Positive predictive value determines how good the test is.

An ideal screening test would have high sensitivity and specificity so that there would be very few false positives or negatives. Yet we know that chest X-rays are not 100 per cent sensitive (that is, as a screening tool, they do not enable 100 per cent of people with tuberculosis of the lungs to be correctly identified; some people with disease are missed). Neither is chest X-ray 100 per cent specific (that is, those without disease might be classified as having disease through screening).

If we assume, from the published evidence, that the sensitivity (the proportion of true cases picked up) of X-ray screening for tuberculosis is 75 per cent and the specificity (the number of true negative cases picked up) is 99 per cent, then we can calculate the probability that an individual for whom the screening test is positive actually has the disease. An example best illustrates the reasons for this.

Chest X-rays are used to screen immigrants from South Africa; the incidence of tuberculosis in new arrivals from South Africa is 600 per 100,000 population. We can calculate the number of cases of disease expected, the number truly identified, and the number with disease who might be missed. If 10,000 immigrants from South Africa were screened, we would expect 60 of these to have disease. But of these 60, only 45 (75 per cent) will have been identified through screening. Moreover, of those 9,940 without disease, about 100 (one per cent) will have been classified as having disease. So, through chest X-ray screening, only 45 out of 145 (31 per cent) individuals identified as having tuberculosis actually have it. This is the positive predictive value. This means that 69 per cent of people classified as having the disease will not, in fact, have it (false positives). In people from countries with lower prevalence rates of tuberculosis the number of false positives will be far greater.

A second example takes the prevalence of 40 per 100,000, the level above which tuberculosis is considered high and the rate at which screening in the United Kingdom is advocated. Of 10,000 immigrants screened, the number of people expected to have the disease would be five; of these, only three (75 per cent) will be identified. But of those 9,995 people without disease, one per cent would be classified as having disease. The proportion of false positives climbs to an astonishing 97 per cent (see Table 6).

Different experts interpret chest X-rays used for screening differently; even the same expert can give a different interpretation on different occasions. In interpreting the same chest X-ray, experts come to different conclusions from those they arrived at previously in about 20 per cent of cases. This may explain why, in screening asylum seekers in the United Kingdom, the number of cases in which tuberculosis was considered to be a possible diagnosis on subsequent review by a different clinician was similar to the number of cases identified on initial screening – that is, as many cases of tuberculosis may have been missed as detected.

Table 6 Results of chest X-ray screening (10,000 immigrants are screened)

Prevalence/ 100,000	Expected no. active cases	Actual no. cases detected	Missed number of cases	False positive cases	True positive cases
600	60	45	15	100	31%
40	4	3	1	100	3%

Extra-pulmonary tuberculosis is much more common (33 per cent) in the new arrivals than in the native population (20 per cent) but extra-pulmonary tuberculosis is not detected on chest X-ray screening.

Notwithstanding doubtful detection of pulmonary tuberculosis by screening with chest X-rays, virtue is made of the much more commonly present healed or quiescent tuberculosis. The abnormalities associated with healed tuberculosis are given prominence to justify use of chest X-rays to screen immigrants. A brief evaluation of this process is provided.

The abnormality most commonly revealed on chest X-rays is past healed or quiescent tuberculosis in asymptomatic people. Healed tuberculosis does not necessarily lead to tuberculosis disease. Most often it will not do so. Experience shows that there is poor compliance with advice on follow-up investigations in these cases. Impact of screening is further reduced when we consider that tuberculosis arising from old infection is characterised by a predominance of patients with disease of minimum extent – lower grade activity, fewer organisms and lesser tendency for the lung lesion to progress for the disease to become infectious. Sputum smear examinations are invariably negative. The immigrants with healed tuberculosis present a relatively higher risk of reactivated disease, but the findings are epidemiologically insignificant, especially as the results would be non-infectious tuberculosis. Besides, in absolute terms the much larger number of immigrants without evidence of tuberculosis will provide the much greater number of cases, and with more pulmonary tuberculosis in the future than people with positive findings in their chest X-rays.

In British Columbia, Canada, out of 21,959 recently arrived immigrants between 1982 and 1985, 1,173 (5.3 per cent) healthy persons were judged to have healed tuberculosis or pulmonary nodule or fibrosis on the basis of chest X-rays. In this group, 1.5 per cent of immigrants were found to have active disease soon after entry; seven further cases arose, giving an average annual incidence rate of 0.33 per cent over a four-year period of study. Similar results were reported in the US during 1975. Among 8,000 persons with previous radiological evidence of healed tuberculosis or pulmonary fibrosis, one per cent developed active disease on arrival or soon after. These rates are much lower than rates obtained subsequently in people who had a clear chest X-ray at the time of entry to the country.

Not only is the value of the procedure doubtful, there are moral and ethical considerations as well, which are explored in the next chapter.

CHAPTER 20

Ethical and Moral Considerations in Screening for Tuberculosis

Global migration has undergone a profound change. There has been an unprecedented explosion of attempts to enter developed countries, by any means, legal or otherwise, in recent years. Monitoring of immigrants, even for the most legitimate reasons of social benefits and housing, let alone screening for tuberculosis, has proved difficult. Legal immigrants are now a part of the immigration pattern. Refugees, asylum seekers, illegal entrants, visitors who do not go back, and students who stay on permanently are the majority who swell the numbers and are likely to escape a screening programme.

Tuberculosis is a curable disease. It is ethical to include immigrants within the tuberculosis control programme on arrival in a host country. The challenge is to treat tuberculosis independently of the person's origin and status in the country.

This is not in dispute. What needs ethical and moral consideration is firstly whether detection needs to begin immediately and involuntarily just before, at the point of, or soon after entry to the country; and secondly if the disease is to be classified and treated differently based on country of origin or race.

The United Kingdom General Medical Council, in its booklet "Serious Communicable Disease", classifies tuberculosis as such and advises that it is not acceptable to test for tuberculosis without the patient's knowledge or agreement. It is for the patient to decide what should be done. Doctors cannot hope to maintain the trust and respect of their patients unless they share information with them, respect their right to autonomy, and trust them as partners in the decision-making process.

The ethical and moral picture has a practical dimension. Compulsion leads to non-compliance with treatment. Considering the deluge of immigrants, legal or illegal, arriving at various ports of entry, spreading all over the country in a short time, adherence with tuberculosis screening control procedures is impracticable. Without voluntary understanding and consent, any measures to control imported tuberculosis would fail unless we turn the whole nation into a police state.

The government is seen to be taking firm, decisive action to bring tuberculosis under control by adopting border control measures to screen immigrants. Occasional detection of cases is highlighted to show positive outcome. This makes screening seem more justifiable and acceptable in the eye of the public.

Yet the effect of measures based on political expediency is ultimately to discourage those at greatest risk of disease from seeking advice and help. This results from the potential for stigma and ostracism that is compounded by the selective tuberculosis screening and detection procedures, in a setting where the immigration process rather than health is the primary concern. It creates an environment in which individuals seek to evade immigration controls, rather than present themselves and remain within the system, for fear of having to overcome another hurdle and being rejected. The consequences are interference in the control of tuberculosis. Important also is the ethical and moral consideration of thousands of radiographs being taken at an airport where quality control can be least expected, because of an unsuitable milieu for communicating with immigrants.

Tuberculosis screening is also a singularly inappropriate medical response in the control of the disease. It serves more to exacerbate, rather than limit, the spread of tuberculosis if false conclusions are drawn, which is not uncommon, or if resources are diverted from effective control programmes. Screening programmes for immigrants to the United Kingdom, despite having been proved to be extremely expensive in terms of results achieved, are difficult to halt once introduced.

We must take into consideration not only the ineffectiveness of screening, but also the unintended consequences that arise from attempts to introduce compulsion into the screening process and the wider public context within which this issue is located. Resources are more effectively channelled into ensuring that all immigrants to the United Kingdom have access to medical care so that tuberculosis is detected promptly and treated appropriately. Only this will guarantee protection against an infectious disease.

Neither can we disregard the issues of consent,

understanding of the need for examination and human rights. The London Heathrow Health Control Unit employs no interpreters. All authorities report non-compliance with referrals of more than 50%, even in countries where compliance is compulsory and supported by law. Once immigrants associate tuberculosis with compulsion and forced investigation, compliance with treatment, which is spread over several months, becomes difficult.

Coercion in screening for tuberculosis is intended to afford protection from transmission of tuberculosis to the host population. This makes sense since identification of those with tuberculosis means that treatment can be initiated and the chain of transmission interrupted. But evidence in support of interruption is absent, and many practical and ethical barriers to the use of coercion present themselves in a free society.

While the author has no evidence that the government in the United Kingdom applies physical or mental coercion in screening for tuberculosis, it does make entry to the country conditional upon consent to be tested. Without consent, new entrants forfeit the right to enter and reside in the country.

The terms coercion, compulsion and conditional screening have political overtones. The author would accept necessity in such matters but does not do so for tuberculosis screening for several reasons. These are that no medical benefits are demonstrated, there is interference with proper controls, costs are prohibitively expensive and resources are diverted from effective programmes. It gives rise to fear and anxiety and discourages people from seeking medical assistance, despite the insistence of the state that no adverse action will be taken against those found to be ill with tuberculosis.

Creating boundaries between groups to prevent the spread of infection has a long historic tradition. Travellers have suffered as a consequence of fears of communicable diseases. Isolation and quarantine are often the first measures called for, but in practice are largely without benefit. Historical analysts have condemned the practice claiming that effectiveness was rarely obvious. What we believe of the infectiousness of tuberculosis is dogma "based on a few scant facts".

Why then do some (all English speaking) developed countries persist with tuberculosis radiological screening for new immigrants?

The reason is political rather than medical. Immigrants bring tuberculosis infection to the host country. Immigrants represent the burden of tuberculosis there. This will continue as long as migration continues from less developed countries. Steps must be taken to prevent the spread of tuberculosis and to protect the host community from contracting illness imported from abroad.

The countries that have introduced screening on entry do not know how to stop "port of entry" screening. The more the screening programmes are shown to be worthless, the more the insistence to continue them to justify their existence.

Doctors and politicians are fearful of infection

overwhelming their population. They want to stop tuberculosis at their frontiers and want something to be done about it. That it is not possible to do so does not detract them from continuing to make demands for it. The false sense of security is preferred instead.

Immigrants bring in the infection and not the disease. Radiological screening will not reveal those persons who only suffer from infection rather than disease.

Taking into consideration the natural decline in the rates of tuberculosis in immigrants once resident in the country, a holding policy, where active cases are efficiently treated and new contacts diagnosed and treated for recent infection, is the most effective way of controlling tuberculosis. A policy of detection and treatment as tuberculosis reveals itself has proved to be the most effective instrument of control in the United States. The United States had the highest rates of tuberculosis anywhere in the developed world until recent years, now it has the lowest – within a decade of adopting the policy of "treat tuberculosis as it presents" instead of seeking it in asymptomatic people as is the case with a screening programme.

CHAPTER 21

Screening: Summing Up

- No evidence that immigrants delay in seeking care for tuberculosis. As long as treatment is provided in time, no spread occurs in the community.

- No evidence that the host population is at risk from immigrant-associated tuberculosis. Tuberculosis in the native-born population is progressing towards elimination by the end of the first quarter of this century.

- Screening programmes fail to reach people such as undocumented immigrants (asylum seekers, illegal entrants), transient workers and visitors who, depending on country of origin, could be at very high risk of tuberculosis. Unstable tuberculosis can lead to disease within weeks of arrival in the country.

- Compulsory screening measures are counter-productive. Those who suspect they may be infected go underground. These measures discourage the very people at greater risk of tuberculosis from seeking care because of fears over the coercive screening. It extends the period of infectiousness and unnecessary transmission to others.

- Professional conduct of health care providers is

compromised if the benefits of compulsory measures are not clearly demonstrable. Public health has a long tradition of resorting to coercive practices, with little evidence of health benefit.

- Tuberculosis control must be rational and coherent to be effective. Screening interferes with control as it mixes effective medical treatment for the sick with competing, irrelevant, programmes for the healthy.

- A "one-off" screening programme will not detect disease in those who travel frequently back to their country of origin where there is a high prevalence of tuberculosis.

- Screening has the perverse effect of creating incentives to avoid timely treatment.

- No evidence exists regarding the benefits of introducing screening for tuberculosis in the country of origin. The data on the links between pre-entry screening and transmission and infection rates in countries of migration has never been made available and most probably does not exist.

- Limited compulsory health screening – for example, of individuals claiming asylum at ports of entry to the UK – will not detect infection in others (for example, in non-port applicants and bona fide immigrant populations). It will lead to a false sense of security that the problem of immigrant-related tuberculosis has been controlled.

- For health screening to be even partly effective in diagnosing tuberculosis, compulsory procedures will have to be introduced for all intending temporary or permanent settlers, visitors, students and job seekers entering the UK, and for all returning British citizens who have lived in a less developed country for a number of years. Native-born nurses, doctors and teachers who have worked abroad are as likely to present with tuberculosis in this country as asylum seekers.

- Changing patterns of global migration will necessitate constant review and change of screening programmes at great cost and disruption to services.

- Determinations of "threshold" of tuberculosis prevalence in a country will mean that large numbers of immigrants from lower prevalence countries will continue to be at risk of disease.

PART SEVEN

Organisation and Management of Services

CHAPTER 22

Organisation of Tuberculosis Contol Services

Organisation requires the following evidence-based factors to be taken into account.

Early diagnosis and treatment

The importance of early diagnosis and treatment of tuberculosis in all patients cannot be overemphasised. Diagnosis of tuberculosis and its treatment within a period following four weeks of disease onset will almost certainly prevent transmission of infection. Transmission of infection indicates treatment failure.

Provided medical intervention is timely, different and enormously varying rates of tuberculosis in native-born persons and those born abroad will respond equally well to treatment, with identical outcomes.

Passive or active management

Do we manage tuberculosis disease as it presents regardless of its antecedents – passive control – or should our knowledge of its natural history lead us to seek out (chest X-ray screening) and treat disease and infection (tuberculin skin test) to protect against spread in the asymptomatic community – active control?

The traditional tuberculosis control programme consists of: passive case finding of self-reporting patients by means of medical history, tuberculin skin test, microscopic examination of sputum, chest X-ray, followed by treatment with standard anti-tuberculosis drugs.

In poor countries, there is no choice, because of lack of resources, but to treat only tuberculosis disease (passive). Active control is beyond their resources. Developed countries may be tempted to provide protection against tuberculosis by active detection and treatment of disease. But should they do so?

The United Kingdom does not have a declared policy of managing tuberculosis but pursues mainly a passive approach to treating disease. The active detection consists only of seeking out recent infection in close contacts of tuberculosis cases and screening of new arrivals to the country.

However attractive an active approach appears, the chance of infection, except in close contacts, ever leading to disease is less than one in 10 over a lifetime.

Early diagnosis, prompt treatment and appropriate follow-up of recent contacts with the disease are the lynchpin of control of tuberculosis. This effectively reduces exposure to tuberculosis in non-infected persons. It leads to the greatest success, as it will control 95 per cent of tuberculosis. In an active programme, to seek out and prevent the remaining five per cent of cases will need immense input of resources far beyond the capacity of any country in the world. Provided tuberculosis in the five per cent population is detected and treated by early diagnosis and treatment, no further spread of the disease will occur.

Active control measures that seek out people with the disease, for example in immigrants, do not measurably add to control of tuberculosis, are not efficient in doing so and are wasteful of resources. However serious tuberculosis is as a disease, prevalence is never high enough, even in countries with rates of tuberculosis 100 to 200 times higher than the United Kingdom, to make active seeking out of cases worthwhile. Moreover, it is not possible to predict which cases of infection will proceed to disease, as only one case in ten will ever do so. Active measures may also create social and political problems when these are directed towards selected segments of the population perceived to be at higher risk of developing tuberculosis than the rest.

It is better to concentrate resources on the most effective measures than spread them thinly and lose the objective of controlling tuberculosis.

Attitude and prejudice

Diseases fade and then return, as has tuberculosis in the developed world. Better housing, nutrition, ventilation, lessening of overcrowding and prohibiting of public spitting are said to have had a slow, but cumulative, secular effect in lowering the prevalence of tuberculosis in the 19th and first half of the 20th century, before the introduction of specific treatment in the developed world in the 1950s, which further dramatically reduced the danger of developing tuberculosis. No such conditions prevail in the less developed world. The population has vastly increased in the past 50 years. It is not possible currently to envisage a steadily enriching, developed world to be duplicated in the less developed world, to bring about similar secular changes in the decline of tuberculosis in the foreseeable future.

While conditions for a decline are not present in the less developed world, tuberculosis spreads not because it is linked to poverty and deprivation but because it is an infectious disease and resources are not available to treat it. It spreads in increasing numbers because there is more, indeed much more, of humanity than ever before. There is relatively more tuberculosis among poor people not because of lack of resistance to disease but because they are deprived of treatment. If treatment were made available, they may still be poor, but they would not be suffering from tuberculosis.

History of disease does not repeat itself, but themes and actions do. Whenever an epidemic occurs, people look for someone or something to blame. Reversal of the trend of tuberculosis in its downward spiral led to the belief, despite evidence to the contrary, that it was due to poverty, deprivation and poor housing in the United Kingdom and that it was inextricably linked to the immigration of people from less developed countries with high rates of tuberculosis.

Illness does not necessarily bring out the best or the rational in humans. Having blamed poverty and deprivation for the persistence of increased prevalence of tuberculosis, the problem has been relatively disregarded as a medical responsibility in the United Kingdom. This is in contrast to the United States where vigorous medical interventions have dramatically reversed the trend from much higher levels than those ever obtained in this country to an expectation of freedom from disease within the next three decades. No such expectation is entertained or even thought of in the United Kingdom. On the contrary, there is an air of pessimism in the face of disease in uncontrolled new arrivals from the less developed world.

An achievement similar to the United States is far from assured in the United Kingdom, though it would be much easier to accomplish. The United Kingdom, after all, boasts of a better, universal, equitable health service available to all those in need, unlike its north Atlantic counterpart. It is interesting to note that Canada, a very rich and much less populated country, next door to the United States, has a similar attitude to tuberculosis as does the United Kingdom and is similarly faltering in its attempt to bring progress of tuberculosis to a halt.

The spread of tuberculosis is for no other reason than transmission from a person suffering from the disease to someone who is not. Other factors may influence transmission, but they do not detract from the fact that interruption of transmission by treating recent infection in close contacts alone will control tuberculosis.

It is not money that is the reason for poor control of tuberculosis – management of tuberculosis is not an expensive commodity – but a commitment to pursue vigorous control based on epidemiological trends of the disease, as clearly demonstrated in the United States where the gap between the rich and the poor is much wider than in this country. The United Kingdom has the additional advantage of offering its citizens universal care, in contrast to the much-derided, divisive medical treatment in the United States that is prohibitively unaffordable by the poor. Yet, it is in the United States that we see a more successful approach to containing tuberculosis than in the United Kingdom.

Medical care differs in both countries but the principles of management of disease do not. Much of what needs to be done is simple and evidence-based. Present expertise relating to tuberculosis is adequate to call an abrupt halt to its spread. So are the available resources for effective control. There is no place for experimentation or a wait and see policy in the control of tuberculosis.

If it is not a question of additional resources – tuberculosis treatment demands so little – then it is a question of attitude change and commitment to the elimination of the disease, rather than the adoption of a fatalistic approach to an easily curable disease.

Tuberculosis is a clinical problem. Treatment of tuberculosis disease and recent infection is simple and easy to perform. The diagnosis is easily made with tuberculin skin testing; basic radiological and laboratory examinations and treatment are effective tools to control tuberculosis. We need no new knowledge or further research to control the disease.

Recent developments in biotechnology are revolutionising

diagnosis, treatment and prevention. But these new tools are useful accessories; they are not essential to eliminate tuberculosis now.

Delay in diagnosis

One of the main causes of failure in treating tuberculosis early is failure of timely diagnosis. Because tuberculosis is now uncommon, doctors often do not consider the possibility of tuberculosis in the diagnosis of disease in a patient.

The total number of tuberculosis cases is low in England. The average general practitioner (GP) will see only about two cases every 10 years. The range will vary widely as some GPs will see several times more cases than others. Numbers will be much higher in areas where people born abroad predominate. It is true to say that even in areas with a large population of people born abroad, the number of cases of tuberculosis seen by a GP will still be low, not exceeding three to five cases annually in very high prevalence areas of London.

Delay in diagnosis has an impact on the individual by increasing the risk of serious illness and death, and unnecessarily increasing risk of transmission. An average delay of 10 to 12 weeks currently takes place before a patient receives treatment for tuberculosis.

Social and economic deprivation

The secular decline in tuberculosis in the pre-treatment era is attributed primarily to improved conditions of living.

The reversal of downward trends in tuberculosis in developed countries in recent years is claimed to be not only due to immigration from high tuberculosis prevalent countries but also to deteriorating socio-economic circumstances of the population, especially for immigrants. For example, in Britain the greatest increase in tuberculosis between 1980 and 1992 occurred in the poorest 10 per cent of the population. In this group, notifications increased by 35 per cent compared with an average national increase of 12 per cent. What this misuse of figures hides is the fact that proportionately more people born abroad live in poor areas. The increase is directly proportional to the number of such people rather than to the number of poor people. There are poor areas in rural counties too but they have little or no tuberculosis.

When tuberculosis is suspected, investigations are carried out, the person is treated and people who are close contacts of the patient are assessed for infection and treated to eliminate such an infection if present. Nothing could be simpler with this medical approach but much misinformation hinders this process from being carried out.

Most authorities on tuberculosis in the United Kingdom insist that it is a disease of poverty and deprivation. No heed is given to the fact that treatment will cure all tuberculosis regardless of unfortunate personal circumstances. If a country, rich or poor, is able to treat tuberculosis promptly and prevent its transmission, again with treatment of recent infection, the disease will be eliminated. No measure of improvement in living standards will eliminate tuberculosis; only medical intervention will do this.

Primary prevention

BCG vaccination has no effect on transmission, and active case seeking in asymptomatic persons by chest X-ray screening does not expose infection and is highly inefficient in detecting disease. Prevention by vaccination and chest X-ray screening of an asymptomatic population has no place in modern management of tuberculosis.

Passive case finding and treatment interrupt the chain of transmission, and treatment of new infection in close contacts of tuberculosis stops infection from progressing into disease. This strategy will lead to successful elimination of tuberculosis in the community.

Epidemiology looks at the determinants and distribution of tuberculosis in the population. It identifies people at high risk of tuberculosis. There is widespread fear relating to tuberculosis in immigrants. There is fear that the higher prevalence of tuberculosis in immigrants poses a threat to the population. Politicians and the medical profession often use immigrants as a self-serving tool to air personal prejudices. The country has responded by screening immigrants at ports of entry at great cost without any noticeable effect on the incidence of tuberculosis. Inflaming prejudice is a self-inflicting wound as it interferes with the subsequent proper control of tuberculosis in the United Kingdom.

Tuberculosis is not transmitted from people born abroad to those born in this country. There is ample evidence of that, supported by irrefutable molecular studies. These findings should help quell the fear that people born abroad are a source of rampant tuberculosis transmission to the native-born population.

Consideration of race has no place in the management of tuberculosis, as genes have no relevance to tuberculosis. Exposure to tuberculosis in a less developed country is a factor of high prevalence of tuberculosis and not a defect in the racial make-up. The same races take on the characteristics of tuberculosis similar to the native-born population after a generation of living in the host country with low prevalence of the disease. Thus Moslems originating from various less developed countries can have a tuberculosis case rate of 2,000 per 100,000 (Somalis) or four cases per 100,000 (Moslems born in this country).

The United States with a poor start a decade ago, with a picture of uncontrolled tuberculosis, has not only managed to control it successfully with medical interventions but has now set targets to eliminate new infection from its entire population.

It is an indictment against the United Kingdom that starting from a very favourable epidemiological picture it still struggles to understand the nature of tuberculosis and fails to come to grips with it.

Risk categorisation

High risk for tuberculosis is a relative concept. The rate of tuberculosis in the United Kingdom-born population is less than four cases per 100,000 population. In the native-born population, examples of high risk are homeless people, drug addicts, people with HIV/AIDS, and prison inmates. Unlike the United States, these categories of people do not form an important segment of the population with risk for tuberculosis, despite their vulnerability to contract the disease. An important reason for this is the social equity and universal availability of health care in the country. Only a tiny proportion of the population escapes the safety net and suffers from social or medical disadvantage.

In the United Kingdom, immigrants from countries with rates of tuberculosis higher than 40 per 100,000 population – an arbitrary rate – are screened for tuberculosis on arrival in the country. The rates are such as to include tuberculosis prevalence in all less developed countries.

Tuberculosis rates in immigrant segments of the population vary enormously from 40 to 2,000 cases per 100,000 population depending on the country of origin of new arrivals. Within the United Kingdom, tuberculosis rates will vary in proportion to rates in the country of origin in different sections of the population. These trends cannot be improved upon by treatment.

The term high risk presents epidemiologically an indefinable amorphous population. What is more important is that even within the high risk population, as within the native-born population with low risk of the disease, the likelihood of infection acquired in the country of origin progressing to disease is five per cent in the first five years of acquisition of infection and another five per cent during the rest of the lifetime – that is 10 per cent in total per individual life time. Numerically disease is more likely to result in segments of population with high rates of imported infection than in those with lower ones, but it will not exceed 10 per cent over an individual lifetime.

An illustration will explain the occurrence of disease from infection imported from a country with a rate of 100 cases per 100,000 population. Five thousand immigrants arrive in the United Kingdom in one year. The number of cases of tuberculosis annually will be five, of which fewer than two would be infectious.

Admittedly, the risk of tuberculosis is much higher in the born abroad group than in the native-born population, but does actively seeking out cases advance the control of tuberculosis proportionately to the effort that will be required?

Much more than even an epidemiological and evidence-based approach to control is the political imperative. How would it be possible to carry out this measure without discrimination and breach of human rights in a segment of the population in a free country?

The concept of high risk is valid in taking into account close contacts of infectious cases, but otherwise it has no place in the management of tuberculosis in the United Kingdom.

The only tuberculosis risk we need consider is the risk of close contacts acquiring infection from a case of tuberculosis. Principles of management are similar in managing both disease and new infection. The aim is to reduce or prevent further exposure of the population to tuberculosis.

Public health factors

A multi-sectoral approach based on advocacy, social mobilisation, community involvement or public health priority is not necessary for successful control of tuberculosis.

The public health approach favours definition of risk factors for tuberculosis, taking into account sex, race and ethnicity, family history, age, and socio-economic status. In non-infectious diseases, lifestyle illnesses, a multi-disciplinary perspective permits the integration analyses of social determinants, geographical and environmental variations, health care access and utilisation, behaviour and lifestyle of individuals, the influence of biopsychology, foetal experience and family history. It suggests that profoundly different actions are required depending upon which level of explanation one focuses upon.

In tuberculosis, to define risk and then carry out an active programme, with considerable investment, for high risk individuals in the form of screening, observation or preventive measures misdirects effort and leaves inadequate resources for the treatment of the small number of people whose infection will progress to disease. This approach may adversely result in greater disease burden in the community. The public health approach has no place in the control of tuberculosis. The medical model suffices.

Age

Tuberculosis in the native-born population is predominantly

a disease of older age and results from reactivation of endogenous infection. Among immigrants it is equally a reactivation, but at all ages. It is spread over the whole population range. Immigrants tend to be much younger in age with fewer elderly people; hence tuberculosis in host countries tends to be concentrated primarily in young adults. Reactivation of old infection is significant in focal geographical areas (with predominance of elderly native-born and immigrant populations) and demographically well-defined populations (elderly and immigrants).

Children and adolescents

Infection in children and adolescents born in the United Kingdom is acquired from an adult and would be of recent origin. Recent infection has 50 times greater chance of developing into disease within one year than an old infection. Tuberculin skin test positive children and adolescents, with their much longer life expectancy, have a high cumulative risk of developing tuberculosis during their lifetime. Children born to immigrant parents are also likely to have infection of recent origin, although this is not always true. For children born abroad, there are two ways that they acquire tuberculosis. It may be recently acquired in this country or it may have been contracted abroad if born outside the country. For reasons of control, infection uncovered during contact examination, whether in a child or adult, is assumed to be recent and always treated.

The emphasis on contact investigation in adults may lead to it being missed in children who are close contacts of an adult with tuberculosis. The only way to find children with tuberculosis, particularly early, is by whole family contact investigation. Since this may be inadequately practised, children with tuberculosis often escape investigation. The family oriented approach improves diagnostic success by not missing close child contacts. A family-centred service makes follow-up easier and more regular.

A firm diagnosis of tuberculosis in children is difficult. It is not always easy to distinguish between disease and infection in children. The disease tends to be generalised and the symptoms are more constitutional than specific. There is no sputum available for bacteriology and radiological findings can be equally non-specific. The diagnosis is most often presumptive, made on epidemiological considerations, including history of contact, rather than clinical evidence.

Tuberculin skin test reactions are not conclusive. A quarter of patients found to have tuberculosis disease have a negative tuberculin skin test reaction. However, for this reason children with symptoms of tuberculosis should always be evaluated for the disease regardless of their skin test results.

Only physicians with experience of tuberculosis in children should be allowed to investigate and treat it. It is one of the most subjective illnesses and there is no place for intuition or guesswork in managing childhood disease.

New (recent) infection

Because about half the risk of developing tuberculosis

disease is concentrated in the first 12 months after acquiring the infection, it is important to detect new infection early. Detection of new infection helps prevent new cases of tuberculosis either immediately or many years later.

Race, ethnicity and geography

Information on race and ethnicity of people with tuberculosis shows that it affects certain racial and ethnic minorities disproportionately. But race and ethnicity are a proxy for geography or country of origin. Indians, for example, refers to both Hindus and Moslems. Moslems from India, Bangladesh, Pakistan, the Middle East and Africa will suffer from high but very different rates of tuberculosis depending on their country of origin. Moslems born in the United Kingdom will have one characteristic difference from Moslems born in any less developed country, that is a very low rate of tuberculosis.

Administering anti-tuberculosis drugs under direct supervision (Direct Observed Treatment – DOT)

Failure of tuberculosis programmes to make an impact on disease rates and development of widespread drug-resistant tuberculosis in less developed countries, owing to mismanaged administration, have led to a change in the policy of drug treatment.

The new approach emphasises improvement of cure rates rather than number of treated patients. Expansion of case finding is pursued only after cure rates are improved. Effective individual case management is the key to be achieved by direct observation of treatment (DOT). DOT is based on the premise that break of transmission is the most important step in controlling tuberculosis. It is more efficient to improve chemotherapy in diagnosed cases than to expand case finding if the results of treatment are poor.

Experience in the United Kingdom shows that provided treatment programmes are effectively conducted, treatment failures are few and it is only necessary for a minority of patients, especially children, to receive treatment under direct observation.

HIV/AIDS

HIV/AIDS prevalence does not affect rates of tuberculosis in the United Kingdom. People with HIV/AIDS suffering from lack of immunity and unable to resist contracting tuberculosis may be expected to influence trends in tuberculosis. There is no evidence of such an impact on tuberculosis in the United Kingdom.

The probability that patients with HIV/AIDS will contract tuberculosis is low because the percentage of individuals aged 20 to 50 years who become infected with tuberculosis is low. The proportion of cases of tuberculosis in patients suffering from HIV/AIDS is relatively high, but the absolute number of these cases will be insufficient to influence the tuberculosis epidemiology. Because of frequent medical attendance, tuberculosis will be detected early enough in these patients for it not to be transmitted to others, even very close contacts or fellow sufferers from HIV/AIDS.

Public education

Awareness campaigns targeted at immigrants have a useful, but limited, role in the control of tuberculosis. Direct patient education aimed at the whole family is more effective. A video film produced for patients and their families has achieved considerable success in an initiative undertaken by the author. The aim is to highlight the warning signs and symptoms of the disease and to explain the importance of compliance with treatment. General public health campaigns directed at unaffected people are undesirable as these lead to alarm and concern in a community not exposed to tuberculosis. A well-conducted contact investigation programme with built-in education is the best tool of public education.

CHAPTER 23

Tuberculosis Control Strategy: Medical Model

Despite problems of unequal care, the success of control of tuberculosis in the United States points to a different management strategy. The tuberculosis epidemic in New York (1985–1992) was classified a medical emergency rather than a public health catastrophe.

The strategy was to treat tuberculosis as an infectious disease and apply medical measures regardless of any public health and social underpinnings. The medical model of tuberculosis management is in contrast to the public health approach to control practised in the United Kingdom – a multi-factor entity requiring complex solutions to its management.

Principles of the medical model

Tuberculosis has a moderately long incubation period. It is difficult to contract. Once contracted, it passes through a long period of infection. If the disease is detected in time, before it has an opportunity to spread, treatment is instituted to make the patient non-infectious. This stops the disease spreading to other people. At least four weeks are available to complete this stage.

If infection does take place, routine contact investigation uncovers it; treatment is again instituted to prevent the infection from progressing further to disease.

Failure to practise the medical model results in the disease progressing to a more serious condition and spreading infection to others. Failure to detect infection results in its accumulation and disease in future. The cycle of tuberculosis repeats itself. The medical model interrupts the cycle and reduces the burden of the disease.

In San Francisco, the tuberculosis prevalence index was seven times higher in US-born blacks than in US-born whites or Hispanics. This difference was not the result of an increased prevalence of human immunodeficiency virus infection or drug resistance among blacks, it was related to historical lack of access to medical care in a marginalised population. The focusing of medical resources on the sub-population in which indices were highest rapidly reduced tuberculosis rates.

From 1991 to 1997, the incidence of recently transmitted cases of tuberculosis in San Francisco, as measured by the number of clustered (indicating outbreaks) cases in the population, decreased substantially, suggesting that the intensification of tuberculosis control measures during this period reduced the spread of infection.

Molecular epidemiology has shown that the links between untreated patients infected with *M. tuberculosis* strains of the same genotype result in accumulation of infected cases over a period of time and lead to apparent outbreaks. This suggests that the outbreaks are due to accumulation of infected cases over a period of time, and not to a linked person-to-person transmission of the same genotype over a unit of time. Again, unlike the pattern of tuberculosis in people in less developed countries, "outbreaks" occur in homeless people, and those in prisons and shelters, because of spread resulting from failure of the treatment programmes. These outbreaks are the result of accumulated cases of infection spread over more than a decade leading to disease – they are not due to active transmission. This is the most likely explanation when outbreaks of tuberculosis are reported in schools, homeless and refugee shelters and prisons.

The failure to practise the medical model has an adverse effect on the incidence of tuberculosis in people who were born abroad. It is to be expected that the children born to such people in this country will be exposed to tuberculosis to a greater extent than the children of native-born parents. This risk is eliminated if the medical model is followed. Detection in time will prevent the disease in adults spreading to their children.

The higher rates of tuberculosis in children born to parents from abroad in the United Kingdom would not occur if focus were placed on a medical model to control tuberculosis.

Persons born abroad are 20 times more likely to develop tuberculosis than those born in the United Kingdom. The distinction in rates of tuberculosis is between being born in the United Kingdom and being born abroad. Many children born in the United Kingdom will be to parents born abroad; prevalence of tuberculosis in this group will be different from that in those born to parents originating in the United Kingdom. Rates vary in the first and, sometimes, in the second and third generations. High rates in people born abroad are unavoidable but high rates in their children and grandchildren are failure of tuberculosis control in the United Kingdom.

UK-born Indian children, for example, have an incidence of 10 cases per 100,000 population as compared with the average prevalence in the United Kingdom born population of four cases per 100, 000 population. But we must compare this with a rate of over 150 cases per 100,000 Indian parents born abroad. Within the same family, an adult born abroad is 15 times more likely to contract tuberculosis than a child born in the United Kingdom. For some adult populations, such as those originating in the African Horn or Central Africa, the risk of developing tuberculosis may be 100 times more than that in their children born in this country. The risk of developing tuberculosis is not related to genes or social conditions but to country of birth of the parents.

The medical model is best suited to a situation where the disease we see today results from infection acquired in the past. Treating the disease stops further spread.

CHAPTER 24

Operational Methodology: Medical Model

The model treats tuberculosis as an infectious disease, curable with anti-tuberculosis antibiotics.

Management is based on a dedicated unit providing family-centred care within a district hospital, with direct access to radiology and microbiology laboratory services. Trained health care workers specialising in tuberculosis operate a tuberculosis unit. Each tuberculosis unit has a minimum number of patients registered at any one time to provide adequate experience in the diagnosis and treatment of the disease.

Objectives

A. Reduce exposure and interrupt transmission from persons with tuberculosis by early detection and treatment,
B. Manage reactivation of tuberculosis infection until the cohorts of infected population pass away with time, and
C. Promptly identify infection in contacts of people with tuberculosis and treat it to prevent progression of infection to active disease.

Goal

Effective early diagnosis, treatment, and prevention of

tuberculosis to achieve zero transmission.

The key to effective control of the disease is diagnosis, which allows prompt detection, especially of all direct sputum smear positive (infectious) cases; and readily-available, efficient chemotherapy regimens, which cure all discovered cases of tuberculosis disease.

Services are delivered from specialised, dedicated centres, maintained, strengthened, and continually evaluated to assure the most beneficial use of available resources.

Targets

1. An incidence of fewer than one case per 100,0000 population born in the United Kingdom, by the year 2025, with an interim target of an incidence of one case per 100,000 population by the year 2010. These are achievable targets and tuberculosis rates are already near this level in UK-born children under five years of age. In some rural areas, tuberculosis has already reached elimination levels. For example in the English Midlands, Hereford and South Staffordshire counties, tuberculosis rates are less than one per 100,000 population.
2. Elimination of tuberculosis transmission in children under 15 years of age to a zero level with immediate effect.

The rates vary in the population, but are low in actual numbers in those born both locally and abroad. Elimination of transmitted disease in the population by treating new infection is an immediate, achievable goal, as the infectious agent is exclusively present in the infected person and is quickly rendered non-infectious with prompt treatment.

In the US, 13 states have reported rates of 1.7 cases, and another nine states 2.7 cases, per 100,000 population. More than half of all states reported no tuberculosis cases in the year 2000.

The pattern of tuberculosis in people born abroad varies depending on the prevalence of tuberculosis in the country of birth and time spent in the host country. Elimination of further tuberculosis transmission in the United Kingdom in those born abroad is also achievable, provided all new infection in contacts of tuberculosis is detected and treated promptly and effectively.

Current problems

Failure of control in the United Kingdom is demonstrated by transmission of tuberculosis, especially in children, from infection acquired in the country. It is a result of:

• Deficiency in identifying and reporting tuberculosis cases and contacts
• Failure to treat recent infection
• Failure of patients to complete prescribed tuberculosis treatment
• Failure to assess the effectiveness of control programmes

- Inappropriate contact investigation
- Lack of sufficient surveillance data to plan services
- Poor delivery of service
- Failure of evidence-based practice of control of tuberculosis

Framework of service

A medically led, specialised, well-defined, nurse-operated management system within a fully integrated clinical service delivery approach is necessary to keep tuberculosis under control.

Modern chemotherapy provides an effective weapon for rapid tuberculosis control The introduction of isoniazid in the early 1950s, followed by pyrazinamide, and the discovery of rifampicin some 20 years later, have allowed for a much shorter period of chemotherapy, administered by mouth, enhancing compliance, and leading to a rapid state of non-infectivity followed by complete cure.

Isoniazid is used for preventive treatment of all child contacts of infected parents and siblings and for secondary treatment of tuberculosis infection in household contacts.

Individual tuberculosis case management provides the central technical strategy. It is devolved through vertical control (categorical or specialised) programmes. These consist of a core structure staffed with specialised personnel at local levels, through which the technical control activities are delivered. This single purpose machinery feeding into the general health infrastructure is developed and managed to provide the specialised delivery service.

Though integration is important, certain aspects of disease control and its technology are hard to incorporate into primary care. However, as gatekeepers, primary care medical practitioners are responsible for initial diagnosis of tuberculosis and referral to the specialised centre. Subsequent primary care responsibility lies in prescribing anti-tuberculosis medication, achieving patient compliance with treatment, and general care of patients in the management of their disease.

Index case referral is the general practitioner's responsibility whereas secondary case finding through contact investigation lies with specialist activity.

The central specialised tuberculosis facility provides service to a defined population segment and has direct access to hospital beds, tuberculosis clinics, X-ray and mycobacterium laboratory facilities; and to contact investigation including tuberculin skin test examination and nurse management teams to conduct clinics and provide supervision of treatment to patients and contacts in the community. There are no specialised hospitals but isolation facilities to treat drug-resistant patients may be required at a national level.

Key functions of a specialised centre are surveillance, monitoring performance, quality, and timeliness. Such a central unit operates through its own allocated resources for training, supervision, logistics, information system evaluation, operational research, and patient health education.

Vertical programmes deliver high cure rates and effectively monitor progress of control efforts. Effective short course chemotherapy, supervision of treatment and rigorous cohort analysis of the treatment outcome need expert management. Vertical programmes become necessary, because of declining trends in the prevalence of tuberculosis, to achieve efficient use of resources and medical expertise. The delivery of the tuberculosis management service in the United Kingdom is already based on a vertical model. The need is to sharpen the focus and deliver an accountable service. Engagement of other sectors beyond health, such as educational and social sectors, in the management of tuberculosis is not necessary.

Components of the programme

Surveillance system: notification registry, treatment surveillance module (monitor treatment progress and outcome, audit morbidity and mortality data, monitor case reporting and case finding procedures, audit quality and completeness of treatment); review progress towards control and the registry for contact investigation.

Training and education: health care workers and the public

Control organisation: management of tuberculosis patients, treatment of recent infected contacts; clinical tuberculosis centres to be linked directly to mycobacterial laboratories to perform mycobacterial cultures; drug susceptibility testing.

For audit purposes, the following module serves as a guide.

Operational structure:

Tuberculosis Unit: A physician cares for 150 patients at any time. Three nurses are attached to each physician for contact investigation and follow-up of contacts until completion of treatment.

Results of positive chest radiographs and sputum specimens are received both by the referral doctor and the tuberculosis unit. Patients with positive sputum specimens are seen within 24 working hours. Patients with positive chest X-ray findings, but negative sputum, are seen within three working days.

Contact investigation is started within 48 hours of a patient starting treatment.

Primary care: Primary care refers a patient with pulmonary symptoms, within three weeks, for a chest radiograph and sputum analysis for tubercle bacilli. If preliminary investigation is negative, and the symptoms persist, a repeat sputum specimen is submitted in three weeks. If the result is negative and the symptoms continue, referral is made to a Tuberculosis Unit.

Following this regime, tuberculosis would no longer be the feared and misunderstood disease it is today, but seen as a straightforward and easily curable condition when dealt with promptly, locally and without political interference.

Postscript

This book was planned and written over the course of five years. I have no reason to believe that much has changed to revise my review of the control of tuberculosis in the United Kingdom. Figures might appear out of date but, unfortunately, even less official information on tuberculosis is available now than in the past. No national annual reports have been published for the years 2003/2004. It should not detract from my argument that a service based on a medical model will bring the spread of tuberculosis to an immediate halt. The recent changes in the national BCG policy, thoughtful readers will by now discern, do not alter my view that BCG vaccination has no place in the management of tuberculosis in the UK.